An Introduction to Acupuncture

It is only when we look to yesterday, today, that we can see tomorrow.

AN INTRODUCTION TO ACUPUNCTURE

A Practical Guide for GPs and other Medical Personnel

Peter Pearson, MBBS, MRCGP, DRCOG

The Medical Centre,
Yateley,
Camberley,
Surrey GU17 7LS

Published in the UK and Europe by
MTP Press Limited
Falcon House
Lancaster, England

British Library Cataloguing in Publication Data

Pearson, Peter
  An introduction to acupuncture: a practical
  guide for GPs and other medical personnel.
  1. Acupuncture
  I. Title
  615.8'92   RM184

  ISBN 0-85200-686-1

Published in the USA by
MTP Press
A division of Kluwer Academic Publishers
101 Philip Drive
Norwell, MA 02061, USA

Printed and bound in Great Britain by Butler and Tanner, Frome and London.

CONTENTS

PREFACE

Several years ago, a patient consulted me, and requested 'aquapuncture'. This sounded more like an underwater sexual activity than anything else, but I confessed ignorance! Several more requests highlighted my complete lack of knowledge of this subject and stimulated me into activity. The public's increased interest in 'alternative medicine', together with a willingness of our trainees to learn about complementary therapies[1] prompted me further.

The purpose of this book is to introduce acupuncture as a practical proposition to busy GPs and related medical personnel. As a concept, acupuncture is understandably rejected by many doctors as being largely devoid of scientific basis and proven benefit. In the form that it is commonly presented, it is often found to be too enormous and unconventional to digest, and also to have too many differing 'schools'.

Here the subject is described very basically, with enough information for the busy clinician to be able to grasp the essentials of traditional Chinese acupuncture and thence, and most important, to be able to practice simple acupuncture on common problems. This latter part is an essential requisite, as without the impetus to actually practise such a discipline at an early stage, many of us would lose interest and confidence, and lose out on feedback from the patients we treat. No dramatic claims are made, but by providing an 'easy opening' to this discipline more clinicians will be encouraged to try it, and then be in a better position to judge for themselves whether the subject is worthy of further study and practice.

Most of this book is devoted to the practical techniques of treating common musculoskeletal problems, which have shown a 60-70% response rate to acupuncture treatment[2-4]. Most of the evidence so far suggests that acupuncture is at least as effective as conventional treatment, but a lot safer. I have purposely dealt only very briefly with the more complex and specialized forms of acupuncture, and take a much simplified approach which I have found effective and easy to learn. The purists will argue that to perform acupuncture at such a simple and local level is at best ineffective and, at worst, harmful. This is nonsense, and I hope to completely dispel this myth. To attempt to learn the whole of traditional acupuncture would in any case be totally impractical for the readers of this book. I have chosen these conditions not only because they are common, but also because they are suitable for this simplified approach. The sufferers of these conditions are often disillusioned with conventional treatments, whether because of poor results or potentially unsafe therapies. Also I feel that there is less 'credibility gap' to be crossed for both clinician and patient.

This book is intended mainly for practising clinicians. A knowledge of conventional medicine is presumed, and indeed mandatory, otherwise the application of what is contained in this book would be impossible. I lay much emphasis on the time element in my approach to acupuncture. The treatment sessions need take no longer than the average GP consultation. Altogether I hope to inspire more clinicians to put into practice, at an early stage, this exciting, safe, and ancient branch of medicine.

ACKNOWLEDGEMENTS

I am indebted to G. Lewith and J. Kenyon who first inspired me, and who taught me most, if not all, I know of acupuncture.

I would like to thank Ralph Davies for drawing the illustrations, and Louise for typing the manuscript (and mastering the physiology of a computer!) and for her many helpful suggestions.

Most of all, I thank my patients, without whom I would never have been able to practice the art of acupuncture.

1
WHAT IS ACUPUNCTURE?

Much of the following chapter will be devoted to the general principles of traditional Chinese medicine. There will be much mind-stretching to say the least! Thankfully, however, the actual amount of information that we need to learn, or even accept, to be able to practise simple acupuncture, is very small indeed. I feel that, despite this, it is necessary to have a grasp of the basic background to acupuncture. This will encompass ideas that are completely new to us, and unacceptable to many. I urge you to treat these as traditional concepts, not to be believed or disbelieved, but to be looked at with an open mind. The science may be wrong but the results may be right.

Acupuncture is a form of therapy that has its origins in traditional Chinese medicine. It has been practised by the Chinese for over 2000 years and was introduced into Europe in 1683 by a Dutch doctor (Willem Ten Rhyme) after a trip to Japan. The earliest references to acupuncture are believed to be in the oldest medical textbook in the world – *The Yellow Emperor's Classic of Internal Medicine*, 300 BC!

The first manuscript detailing the art was written about 200 BC: *Huangdi Nei Jing*. Legend has it that acupuncture was first discovered by a soldier shot by an arrow, who found that when struck by a second arrow, this relieved the pain from the first. Acupuncture is therefore probably the oldest surviving medical discipline, and this surely begs the thought "there must be something in it".

Traditional Chinese medicine described channels (or meridians) in the body, which, although internal, can be mapped out on the body surface for the purposes of identification. Along these channels flows 'qi' – otherwise known as 'vital energy'. At this stage, understand that qi is a concept, and not an identifiable substance.

In a similar vein (sorry about the pun), there is no anatomical or physiological basis for the channels. Another concept is the 'Yin–Yang balance'. The Yin forces are negative in nature and the Yang, positive. Good health exists when these forces are in equilibrium. Imbalance of Yin–Yang causes disease, and this is reflected by a disordered flow of *qi* in one or more channels. By inserting needles (or other stimuli) in certain points along these channels, the flow of *qi* can be corrected and so restore the body to a normal Yin–Yang balance.

There are twenty-six channels in all, twelve pairs and two midline. Out of the twelve, six end in the upper limbs and six end in the lower limbs. These dozen channels are named after organs, whose functional activities are (partially) reflected in the corresponding channels. The organs described in traditional Chinese medicine have functions very much wider than in conventional medicine. I will describe these functions briefly later in this chapter for the sake of completeness, although they have little bearing at this stage. However, if only for purposes of identification, the channels have been named in the traditional manner (Table 1).

Table 1 The channels

Channel	Yin/Yang	Position
Lung, Heart, Pericardium	Yin	Upper limb
Large intestine, Small intestine, *Sanjiao*	Yang	
Spleen, Liver, Kidney	Yin	Lower limb
Stomach, Urinary bladder, Gall bladder	Yang	
Du		Midline posterior
Ren		Midline

The reference to whether the channel is Yin or Yang in nature is, again, not vital to us. Each organ is described as either 'Zang' (the corresponding channel then being Yin) or 'Fu' (Yang channel).

We are not finished yet! According to traditional Chinese medicine, there are certain 'pathogens' that can invade and become important in the causation of disease. The traditional pathogens are as follows: heat, cold, wind, damp, phlegm. We can certainly understand some of these (heat, cold, damp) when applied conventionally to certain rheumatological diseases, but on the whole our minds are stretched once more! Once again, this is not vital to us. Suffice it to say at this stage that there are various acupuncture points described which are supposed to disperse these pathogens (Chapter 6). The other types of pathogen, collectively known as the 'social pathogens', we can all understand: diet, exercise (lack of or excess), pollution, poisons, trauma. These are familiar enough to us in conventional medicine.

As promised earlier, I will now summarize the main functions of the organs, as described in traditional Chinese medicine:

Heart: Dominates the circulation of blood. Keeps the mind healthy.

Liver: Maintains the free flow of blood and qi through the body.

Spleen: Governs digestion and blood. Maintains muscle bulk.

Lung: Controls respiration and the passage of water. Dominates the hair and skin.

Kidney: Dominates growth and reproduction. Produces marrow. Controls body water.

Pericardium: As in conventional medicine

Sanjiao: Otherwise known as the three cavities or the triple warmer organ. No apparent copnventional equivalent. Seems to encompass areas in the chest, epigastrium, and hypogastrium. Functionally controls body temperature.

The following organs seem to have similar functions to their conventional equivalents: small intestine, gall bladder, stomach, large intestine, urinary bladder.

Traditional Chinese diagnosis of systemic disease, caused by organ dysfunction and pathogen invasion, involves eliciting special signs that are completely foreign to conventional medicine.These include pulse changes and various tongue appearances. The concepts involved in diagnosing and treating systemic disorders will be discussed more fully in Chapter 6.

What are we to make of all this? You have been patient to read this far and not throw up the book in horror, banishing any thought of ever practising acupuncture! All I have tried to do, up to this stage, is give you a brief synopsis of some of the principles of traditional Chinese medicine.

You could easily discard all this, and still practise simple acupuncture, as I hope to show you in the next chapter. However, I feel it is important to have the basic background information, however incredible, before we can make the choice of how we are going to get started.

As in all these fringe disciplines, we need a simple opening, for there is too much that is incredible, complex, or just lacking in sufficient scientific basis. The only concept that I would like you to hang on to at this stage, is that of the *channels*. These can be mapped on the body surface (Chapter 3) but lie anywhere from subdermal to three inches from the surface, depending on the position.

The most simple form of acupuncture is treating what the Chinese term *local dysfunction of channels*, which amounts to common musculoskeletal conditions. Local dysfunction implies that pathogens or organ pathology play no part in the pathogenesis or treatment of these conditions, but in traditional teaching this is far from the truth. However, be assured that for our purposes, these conditions are highly amenable to simple acupuncture at a local level. So without further ado, let us get started!

2
LOCAL DYSFUNCTION OF CHANNELS

This chapter deals with acupuncture at its simplest and in many respects is the ideal way to get started. We can, for the moment, leave aside the ideas of pathogens and organ pathology, and concentrate on conditions that, according to traditional Chinese teaching, are caused and correctable by a purely localized disordered flow of *qi* involving one or more channels. The majority of common musculoskeletal conditions that we see fall into this category, and are ideal for this approach.

Precise, conventional diagnosis is not important for this method. This idea will come easily to practising GPs but not to some other medical personnel. However, a paramount principle is that all serious, or potentially serious, pathology should be excluded before embarking on any acupuncture treatment. This, I am sure, is second nature to us as conventional doctors, but more difficult, if not impossible, for the lay practitioner. The conditions tend to fall into three broad categories: the soft tissue rheumatisms (tenosynovitis, epicondylitis, shoulder–neck problems, etc.), chronic or recurrent pain (low back pain being the most common) and acute musculoskeletal pain. The first two categories are the best to treat in a GP setting. Conventional treatment of the first commonly involves local steroid injection with its inherent risks. Patients belonging to the second category have often been 'through the mill' with unsatisfactory results – at best "there is nothing more I can do for you"; at worst, side effects from conventional therapy.

The principle of acupuncture treatment of these disorders is the use of *local and distal acupuncture points*. One firstly identifies the site(s) and radiation of the pain. The patient is then carefully examined for tender points. These have their conventional equivalents (trigger points, fibrocystic nodules), and are often very specific for certain conditions: the lateral epicondyle in tennis elbow, and the subacromial bursa in subacromial bursitis. In other conditions, they will take some painstaking searching (literally!), but they will always be found, often on points along channels. These points will become more familiar with experience, and found very quickly in certain conditions. The tender points are termed *ashi*. The other types of local points, I term *key points*. These are traditional acupuncture points found, by experience, to be useful in certain conditions, whether or not they be tender. These will be described later in this book, when the more specific conditions are dealt with.

Now for the *distal points:* the concept of distal points is much more difficult for us to comprehend and accept. Each of the channels have key distal points, which, according to traditional teaching, it is at least as vital to treat as the local points, in order to execute any change within that channel. Note is made of the channels involved, not only with the *ashi*, but also with the site of pain, *and radiation*. The distal points of those channels are then the points to select. These points will be described in detail in Chapter 3. The use of distal points causes as much incredulity to the patients as to the practitioners – sticking a needle in a foot for pain in the neck will stretch the most open mind! Nevertheless, this is traditional teaching, and forms part of this basic approach. Most of the studies that have attempted to evaluate the effectiveness of acupuncture treatment of painful conditions use this technique [4]. However, it has to be said that there are other views on this subject – including the use of tender points only; but these are too 'modern' to be considered in this type of book at the present.

Let us then recap this method of treatment. The tender points are found by careful examination. Any key local points are noted. The channels are then identified on which lie the following: tender points, site of pain, site of radiation. The distal points of these channels are then noted. The points to treat will therefore consist of: tender point(s), key local points (if any), appropriate distal point(s). In practice, there will be many occasions when the *ashi*, pain and radiation all lie on one or two channels, and hence make the selection of points very simple.

At this stage, many of you will (I hope!) be raring to go, but, alas, we have a little more learning to do. The *ashi* will be simple enough to find, after a little practice, but we need to know the positions of the channels and their respective key and distal points. The next chapter will deal with this and then look into actual practical technique.

3
THE CHANNELS AND POINTS

In Chapter 1, I dealt briefly with the nature and names of the channels. Table 1 will remind us that there are twelve pairs ending in either upper or lower limbs, and two midline channels. We will keep to the conventional names of channels despite the fact that you may well be sceptical of the apparent association of organ-named channels and systemic functions. As we have seen, for the method described in Chapter 2, this concept does not have to be accepted but it is useful to have some knowledge of it if one ventures further into the acupuncture treatment of systemic disease (Chapter 6).

The channels can be conveniently mapped on the body surface in the form of lines. These will be demonstrated diagrammatically and described in turn, together with the surface location of respective key points. Further details of depth (and directional aspects) of channels and points will be given in Chapter 4.

The naming of points is steeped in tradition! I will keep to the straightforward method of naming by channel and a number. In more traditional teaching, each point has a name (in Chinese) but this is obviously more difficult to remember. When one also considers that over one thousand points are described in traditional books, it is no wonder that Western doctors are put off! Thankfully, it is not necessary to learn all these points. For our purposes, it is only necessary to learn the location of a few local and distal points and the channels themselves.

The positioning of the channels and points uses anatomical landmarks and a rather special measurement called the *cun*. Is it not sensible, and more accurate, to use a personal measurement, rather than a conventional one, when locating a point on the body surface? In their infinite wisdom, the Chinese recognized this and hence the *cun*. The *cun* is the maximum diameter across the interphalangeal joint of the *patient's* thumb, i.e. the widest bit of the thumb. On average, it is about an inch, but obviously varies from patient to patient.

THE LARGE INTESTINE CHANNEL

The large intestine channel runs from the index finger, along the antero-lateral aspect of the upper limb, and ends on the contralateral side of the face, close to the nose (Figure 1).

KEY LOCAL POINTS

L.I.15: at the anterior, inferior border of the acromioclavicular point.

L.I.14: at the lower end of the deltoid.

L.I.11: midway between the lateral epicondyle and the lateral end of the cubital crease.

DISTAL POINTS

L.I.11: as above.

L.I.4: in the centre of the triangle between the first and second metacarpals and margin of web (dorsal aspect).

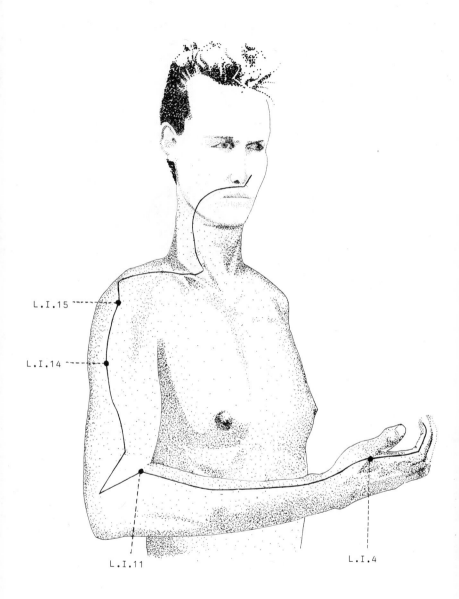

L.I.15

L.I.14

L.I.11

L.I.4

Figure 1 The large intestine channel

THE SMALL INTESTINE CHANNEL

The small intestine channel runs from the little finger, along the postero-lateral aspect of the upper limb, around the scapular region and ends in front of the ear (Figure 2).

DISTAL POINT

S.I.3: proximal to the fifth metacarpo-phalangeal joint, at the end of the transverse crease (palmar surface).

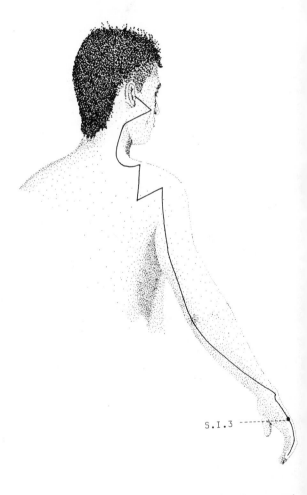

Figure 2 The small intestine channel

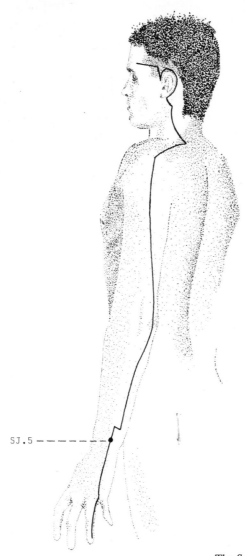

SJ.5 -------

Figure 3
The *Sanjiao* channel

THE *SANJIAO* CHANNEL

The *sanjiao* channel runs from the ring finger, along the lateral aspect of the arm, between the small and large intestine channels. It ends just lateral to the eye (Figure 3).

DISTAL POINT

S.J.5:   2 *cun* above the wrist crease, between the radius and ulna.

19

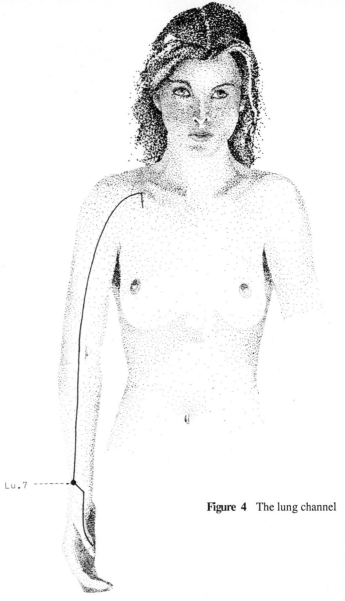

Lu.7

Figure 4 The lung channel

THE LUNG CHANNEL

The lung channel runs from below the clavicle, along the medial aspect of
the arm, through the cubital fossa, and ends in the thumb (Figure 4).

DISTAL POINT

Lu.7: 1.5 *cun* proximal to the wrist crease, medial aspect of radius.

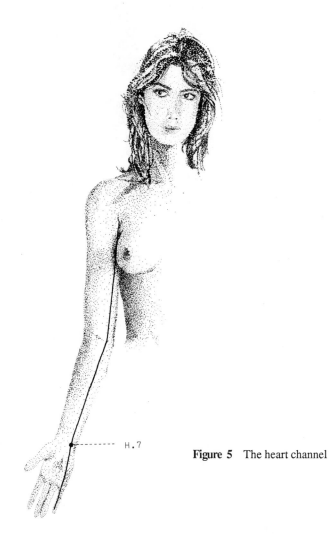

Figure 5 The heart channel

THE HEART CHANNEL

The heart channel starts in the axilla, runs along the postero-medial aspect of the arm and ends in the little finger (Figure 5).

DISTAL POINT

H.7: ulnar side of wrist crease, between head of ulna and the tendon of the flexor carpi ulnaris.

21

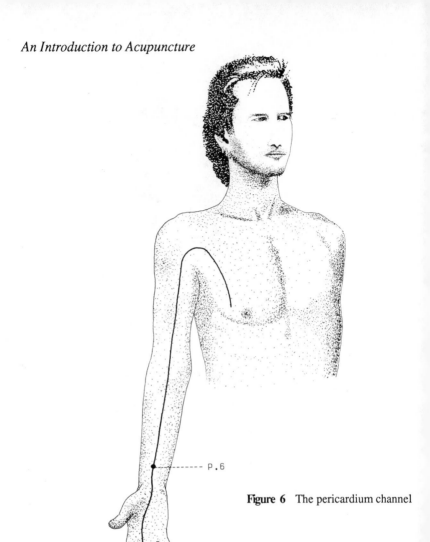

P.6

Figure 6 The pericardium channel

THE PERICARDIUM CHANNEL

The pericardium channel starts lateral to the nipple, runs along the medial aspect of the arm between the lung and heart channels and ends in the middle finger (Figure 6).

DISTAL POINT

P.6: 2 *cun* above wrist crease, between the tendons of palmaris longus and flexor carpi radialis.

THE STOMACH CHANNEL

The stomach channel starts on the side of the face, runs along the side of the chest and abdomen, and down the anterior surface of the lower limb to end in the second toe (Figure 7).

KEY LOCAL POINTS

St.35: in the depression, just below and lateral to the patella.
St.31: directly below the anterior superior iliac spine, level with the lower border of the pubic symphysis.

DISTAL POINTS

St.36: 3 *cun* below inferior border of patella, 1 *cun* lateral to tibia.
St.44: in web between second and third metatarsophalangeal joints, just anterior to those joints.

THE URINARY BLADDER CHANNEL

The urinary bladder channel starts above the eye, passes posteriorly round the scalp and descends down the neck and back. It divides into two lines from the posterior hairline: one line goes down 1.5 *cun* lateral to the midline of the back; the second, 3 *cun* lateral. The channel then descends along the posterior aspect of the lower limb, the lateral aspect of the ankle and foot and ends in the fifth toe (Figure 8).

DISTAL POINTS

U.B.40: in centre of popliteal fossa.

U.B.60: midway between the lateral malleolus and tendo achilles.

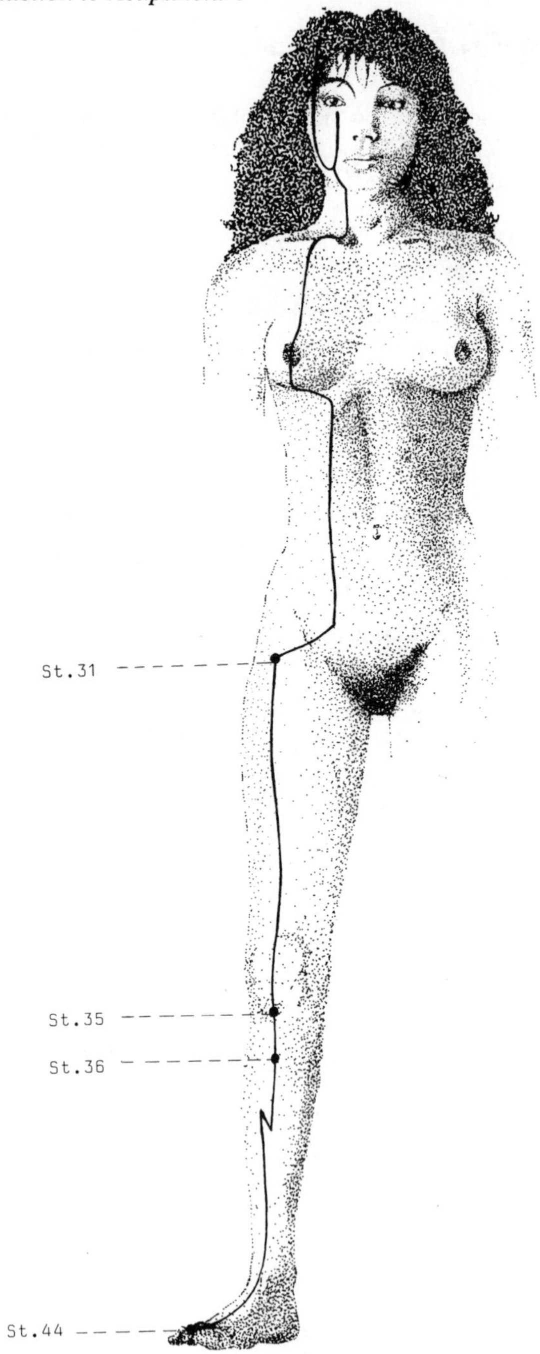

St.31

St.35

St.36

St.44

Figure 7 The stomach channel

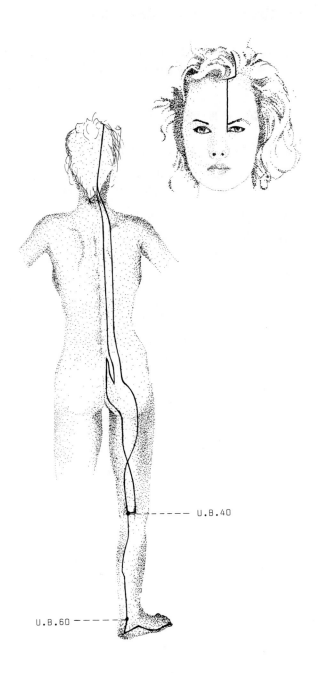

Figure 8 The urinary bladder channel

THE GALL BLADDER CHANNEL

The gall bladder channel starts lateral to the eye, passes through the lateral side of the head, trunk and lower limb, and ends in the fourth toe (Figure 9).

KEY LOCAL POINTS

G.B.8: 1.5 *cun* above the point of the ear (taken when folded over).

G.B.19: midway between the superior border of the occipital protuberance and the superior border of the mastoid.

G.B. 14: 1 *cun* above the midpoint of eyebrow.

G.B.20: half way along a horizontal line joining the inferior border of the mastoid to the midline.

G.B.21: midway between the spinous process of T1 and the acromion.

G.B.29: midway between the anterior superior iliac spine and the greater trochanter (Lateral aspect).

G.B.30: at the junction of the outer third and inner two thirds of a line between the greater trochanter and the sacral hiatus.

DISTAL POINTS

G.B.34: in the depression anterior and inferior to the head of the fibula.

G.B.40: in the depression anterior and inferior to the lateral malleolus.

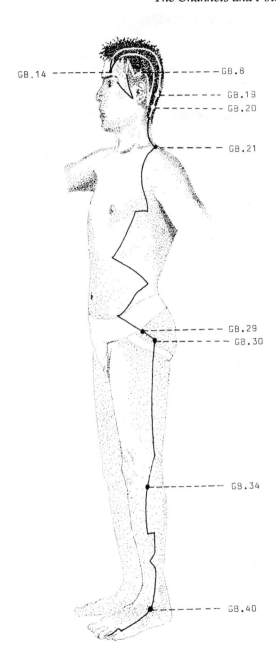

Figure 9 The gall bladder channel

THE SPLEEN CHANNEL

The spleen channel starts in the great toe, runs along the antero-medial aspect of the lower limb and the side of the abdomen, and ends at the top of the chest (Figure 10).

KEY LOCAL POINT

Sp.9: on the inferior border of the medial condyle of the tibia, just posterior to the tibia.

DISTAL POINT

Sp.6: 3 *cun* above the tip of the medial malloeolus.

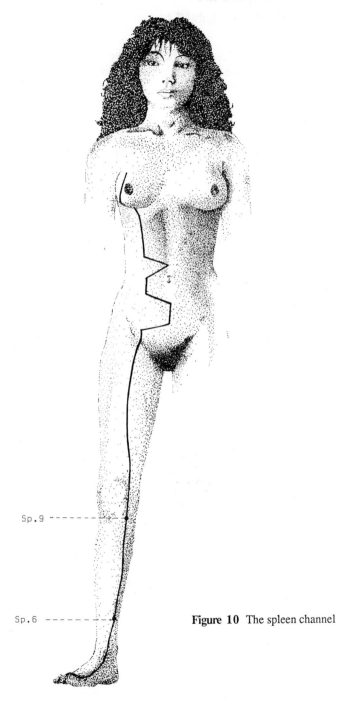

Sp.9

Sp.6

Figure 10 The spleen channel

THE KIDNEY CHANNEL

The kidney channel starts on the sole of the foot, ascends along the postero-medial aspect of the lower limb and the side of the abdomen, and ends at the top of the chest (Figure 11).

DISTAL POINT

K.3: midway between the tip of the medial malleolus and tendo calcaneus.

THE LIVER CHANNEL

The liver channel starts on the great toe, ascends along the medial aspect of the lower limb and the lateral aspect of the abdomen, and ends in the chest (Figure 12).

DISTAL POINT

Liv.3: between the first and second metatarsals, posterior to the first metatarsophalangeal joint.

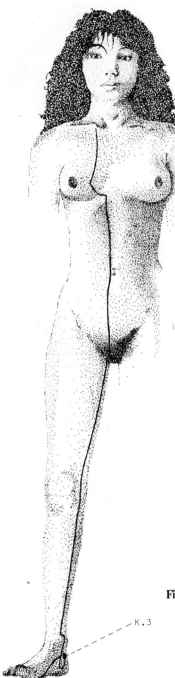

Figure 11 The kidney channel

K.3

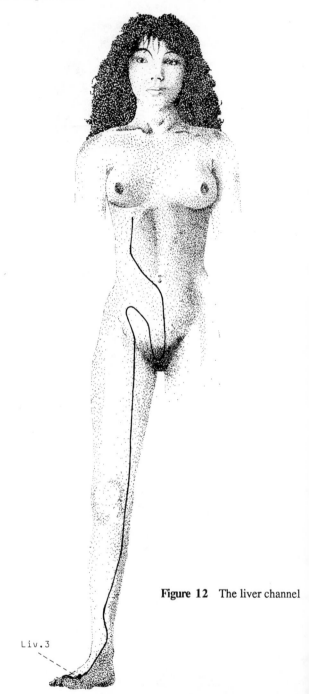

Figure 12 The liver channel

Liv.3

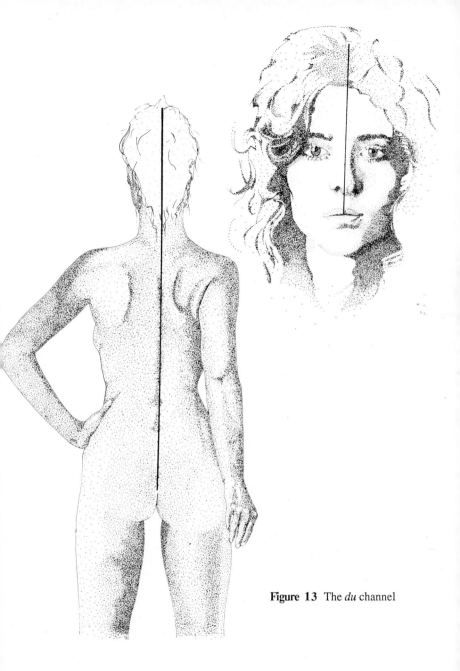

Figure 13 The *du* channel

THE *DU* CHANNEL

The *du* channel starts below the coccyx and ascends along the midline of the back, head and face, and ends in the upper lip (Figure 13).

THE *REN* CHANNEL

The ren channel starts in the centre of the perineum, ascends along the midline of the abdomen, chest, and neck, and ends just below the lower lip (Figure 14).

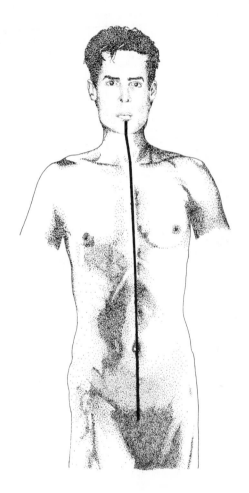

Figure 14 The *ren* channel

Table 2 summarizes the channels and their respective key and distal points.

Table 2 Channels and important points

Channels Key	Local points	Distal points
Large intestine	L.I.15, L.I.14, L.I.11	L.I.11, L.I.14
Small intestine		S.I.3
Sanjiao		S.J.5
Lung		Lu.7
Heart		H.7
Pericardium		P.6
Stomach	St.35, St.31	St.36, St.44
Urinary bladder	G.B.8, G.B.14, G.B.19, G.B.20, G.B.21, G.B.29, G.B.30	G.B.34, G.B.40
Spleen	Sp.9	Sp.6
Kidney		K.3
Liver		Liv.3

It is obviously easier to visualize the location of the channels by means of a body model with the channels marked on it. Such models are available from suppliers of acupuncture equipment (Chapter 9). I would urge you to purchase one.

You will have noted that certain channels have more than one distal point described – really it is a matter of personal choice or anatomical convenience depending on the position of the patient. The key local points are all useful in certain conditions and disease areas. They will be specifically demonstrated in Chapter 5.

A large proportion of musculoskeletal pains (including sites of radiation) occur on the 'outer' surfaces of the body (i.e. lateral, anterior and posterior aspects). This corresponds more to the Yang channels (large intestine, small intestine, *sanjiao*, stomach, urinary bladder, gall bladder) and, by implication, are therefore more important to familiarize oneself with when using the 'local and distal point' technique. In contrast, it is interesting that the Yin organs (and corresponding channels) seem to have more important systemic influence with regard to treating systemic disease; but this is far beyond the principles of purely local acupuncture. Chapters 5 and 6 will, however, include treatment of some systemic illnesses for the benefit of those who feel they are willing to try this sort of acupuncture treatment.

Many acupuncture points will be found in natural 'depressions' including *ashi*. In fact, a relatively modern view is that there is a demonstrable descreased skin resistance over acupuncture points, but this, I feel, is taking it too far. However, it is useful to bear this in mind on certain occasions when difficulty is experienced in point locating.

We now have the principles of local and distal point treatment and have looked at the channels and their relevant key and distal points. Some of you, no doubt, can already visualize these points on some of your patients and are itching to stick any old pin in the same! But it is not 'any old pin, any old size and any old direction', which brings us neatly to Chapter 4. This deals with technique in its widest sense. After reading this chapter, you will be ready to put into practice all the foregoing theory that you have been patient enough to assimilate.

4
TECHNIQUE

Acupuncture treatment consists of inserting needles into acupuncture points, thereby stimulating some sort of change within those areas and channels. Needling is the most traditional method of point treatment and still regarded as the most satisfactory, despite competition from a lot of other more modern treatment methods. These include electrical, laser, or just manual pressure, and will be discussed in Chapter 7. Provided certain precautions are taken, needling is safe and relatively atraumatic (even to the most needle-phobic, myself included!). This chapter will deal with all the necessary detail needed for satisfactory needling technique.

NEEDLES

The main requirements of an acupuncture needle are a sharp point, narrow gauge (28 or finer) and a handle/grip of some sort. Their fineness ensures a relatively pain-free entry and minimal risk of bleeding after withdrawal. The standard needle is made of stainless steel and is re-usable (after proper sterilization). Other metals are used, including gold and silver, but this is for more specialized use and need not concern us here. Handles can be variously specified as coil or spiral, but again this is not important for our purposes.

Acupuncture needles come in various lengths, the most commonly used being half-inch, one-inch, one-and-a-half inch, and three-inch. (The latter size, you will be relieved to hear, is only used for one point where there is plenty of protection!). The one inch size is the most often used but all acupuncture points have different needle size requirements which will be shown later in this chapter.

A relatively modern innovation is the availability of disposable needles and these, to my mind, are the ideal. 100% sterility and sharpness are guaranteed but they are of course more expensive. Some of these have non-metallic handles which, although more comfortable to manipulate, deny the ability to attach electrodes to them for electrical stimulation (Chapter 7). As I have hinted earlier on, this is not a major drawback. I would recommend the use of disposable needles for acupuncture.

NEEDLE INSERTION

If you try to poke an acupuncture needle in like an ordinary hypodermic needle, you will end up with a bent needle, an upset patient and an embarrassed operator! The correct way of holding an acupuncture needle is by gripping the handle between thumb and forefinger and steadying the shaft with the middle finger (Figure 15).

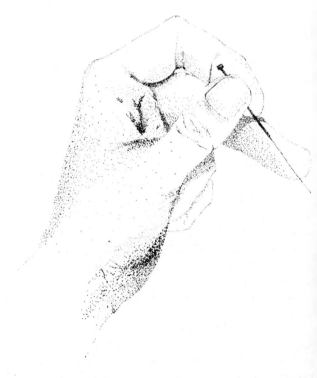

Figure 15   Inserting an acupuncture needle

The skin of the required point is punctured smartly and the needle pushed home to the required depth, in the right direction (see later). By constantly using the middle finger as a support and applying the insertion pressure directly down the axis of the needle, bending and breakage will be avoided. This applies especially to the longer lengths. With the three-inch size, the needle should be gripped low down the shaft for the initial puncture. Thereafter, 'feeding in' the needle can be done either using one hand, as above, or both hands employing the thumbs and forefinger of one as the support. It really is quite easy after a bit of practice but experimenting on an orange, using the above techniques with the different size needles, is to be recommended!

It is *not* necessary to swab the skin before treatment; as you are well aware, doubts have been raised in conventional medicine about the usefulness (or lack of it) of skin swabbing prior to injections etc. It would not therefore surprise you to learn that infection secondary to acupuncture treatment is very rare indeed. Normal hygiene, cleanliness and adequate needle sterility are probably the most important factors.

I make no apology for mentioning reassurance. Most of your patients will naturally be nervous, and some frankly terrified. A good manner will go a long way to obviating the above aspects. Due to the fineness of the needles and (it is hoped!) the skill of the operator, acupuncture needle insertion should *not* be a painful experience.

A brief word about needle withdrawal – the withdrawal pressure should again be applied in the axis of the needle, to avoid breakage and lessen discomfort. Bleeding only occasionally occurs (even in 'hot spots' like U.B.40) and then should be stopped smartly with firm pressure from thumb or swab on the puncture site to lessen the risks of bruising or haematoma formation. The comparative rarity of any bleeding problems owes itself to the relative fineness of acupuncture needles.

NEEDLE MANIPULATION

Once a needle is inserted into an acupuncture point, a certain sensation called *'deqi'* has to be experienced by the patient before any therapeutic benefit is achieved. According to traditional teaching, this is of paramount importance and furthermore is unlikely to occur if the needle is not accurately located.

Deqi is variously described as a deep soreness, aching, burning, spreading or tingling sensation, not only in the area of puncture, but frequently up and down the particular channel. To achieve this, the needle is manipulated in a certain way until that sensation is felt by the patient. The best method is a combined rolling back and forth of the handle between thumb and index finger, together with a simultaneous up and down movement of the needle (Figure 16).

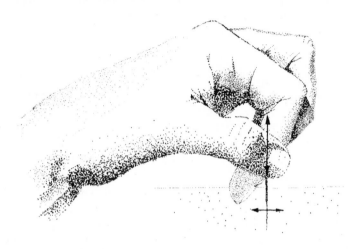

Figure 16 Manipulating an acupuncture needle

Although *deqi* is uncomfortable, it should not be very painful (apart from certain points which are not advocated in this book). A superficial pricking sensation is not *deqi*. If this occurs the needle may be slightly withdrawn and re-inserted at a different angle or depth until needle stimulation has produced the desired *deqi*. This often only takes a few seconds but sometimes takes up to a minute to achieve. Once *deqi* is experienced, there is no virtue in continuing to stimulate and the needle should just be left *in situ*. Traditional teaching on this subject is most complex in that certain conditions need certain points to be highly stimulated and other points 'sedated' or 'reduced' (less stimulated). I would say at this stage that this is unimportant and the technique described above would suit all the methods advocated in this book.

Some patients (low reactors) take a fair amount of needle stimulation to achieve *deqi* and conversely others (high reactors) may experience extreme *deqi* more or less immediately and even while the needle is immobile. These high reactors should certainly not be stimulated further, and needles should only be left in for a comparatively short time. Nowhere is *deqi* more important to achieve than in the *ashi* – the patient will be able to tell you that you have 'hit the right spot'. When treating *ashi* in acute soft tissue pain, adequate stimulation will often result in a local anaesthetic action – much to the pleasure of the patient and the satisfaction of the clinician.

There is no scientific explanation for *deqi*. Again, we have to accept a traditional principle that seems fundamental to successful acupuncture. I would certainly say that in my own experience, when I have not produced *deqi*, the patients have usually not responded to treatment.

When using a conventional steroid injection into a tennis elbow, the old adage that "you are not in the right place until it hurts" has some bearing here – although I hasten to add that acupuncture treatment of the same condition is a good deal less painful!

DEPTH AND DIRECTION

Alas, a little more learning is necessary before progressing further. We have learnt that the channels depicted on the body surface only mark the point of entry for an acupuncture needle. The actual point to be treated will lie a variable depth and direction beneath the skin surface. We need to know two things after choosing and locating the point : firstly the size of the needle to use, and secondly the direction of insertion.

Ashi in conditions such as tennis elbow and subacromial bursitis will be familiar enough to us in conventional medicine. One should end up in the same place as when giving a steroid injection. In the above two examples, putting a one inch needle in, either obliquely or perpendicular to the skin surface, to arrive at the right point would be correct. The production of *deqi* would furthermore confirm the proper location. It would sometimes be more appropriate, especially in a thin person, to use a half-inch needle in some tennis elbow and tenosynovitis *ashi*. Experience, personal preference and individual patient variation will often play a part in needle selection. The important thing is that the right point is hit.

It is impractical (and probably unnecessary) for us to be too dogmatic about point location. To argue, for example, that each acupuncture point may be in an area smaller than a pinhead is academic (and rather awesome!), provided one accepts the principle of *deqi*. If *deqi* is produced with the *ashi* and traditional points, it is fair to assume that the needle is properly located. To simplify matters further, I will firstly describe some fairly broad generalizations and then more specific acupuncture points.

GENERALIZATIONS

The most popular size of needle is the one-inch. This will suit more than 50% of points, not only for anatomical reasons, but also for its ease of handling. One can always vary the depth and direction to achieve the right location.

For the face and scalp, a half-inch needle is the most appropriate. Insert obliquely and just subcutaneously to arrive at the right point – inserted perpendicularly they have a tendency to fall out!

In the neck, shoulder regions, and upper limbs, a one-inch needle is usually required (except G.B.21 and L.I.14 – see next section). The total depth and direction is often governed by anatomical factors. When needling *ashi* above the scapula, for example, gradually increase the depth of insertion until *deqi* is produced, preferably well before hitting the pleura! The same applies to the chest and abdomen, regarding the pleura and peritoneum, respectively.

The most common *ashi* on the back will be found to lie on the U.B. channels. Remember that there are two divisions to this channel – one positioned 1.5 *cun*, the other 3 *cun*, lateral to the midline. The appro-priate needle is the one-and-a-half inch (one-inch for thinner subjects). The direction of insertion is obliquely (45 degrees to the skin surface), towards the midline (medially).

Around the hip and buttocks lie a lot of key traditional points which will be detailed in the next section. Apart from these, a one-and-a-half inch size needle will be most often used.

In the lower limbs, a one-inch needle would be more often used, apart from in the obese, and St.36 (see next section).

If in doubt, use a one-inch needle and go in perpendicularly. The production of *deqi* will tell you that you are in the right place.

SPECIFIC POINTS

If a particular point is not mentioned in this section, applying the above guidelines will cover most eventualities.

L.I.14: insert one-and-a-half inch needle posterior to the lower end of the deltoid - direct the needle antero-medially in the horizontal plane.

L.I.4: use a one-inch needle, obliquely towards apex of 'triangle'.

S.I.3: one-inch needle, perpendicularly to medial edge of hand, to pass in front (palmar aspect) of fifth metarcapal.

St.36: one-and-a-half-inch needle, directed downwards and medially.

G.B.20: one-inch needle in a direction towards the opposite eye.

G.B.21: one-and-a-half-inch needle (one-inch in thinner subjects), di-rected anteriorly, but in a horizontal plane (avoids the lung apex!)

G.B.30: the only point in this book using a three-inch needle, directed towards the opposite hip.

FURTHER GUIDELINES ON TREATMENT

We have reached the stage of point selection and identification, employing the correct size needle, inserting the same in the proper direction, and then producing *deqi*. The remainder of this treatment session consists of leaving the needles *in situ* for five to ten minutes, and then a little more needle manipulation to produce *deqi* just prior to withdrawal. It is wise, incidentally, to have the patient on a couch throughout treatment – not only to encourage relaxation, but also to lessen the risk of fainting. It also pays to have a sympathetic helper to talk to the more nervous patients during the treatments, especially the first one.

It can be seen that by employing the above method, one can easily treat patients in the middle of surgeries with little disruption. Having a clinic set aside for acupuncture lends itself to being able to treat large numbers of patients at once – provided there are sufficient rooms available! It may literally only take seconds to insert the needles and produce *deqi*, and then one simply proceeds to the next patient.

In a general practice setting, I would advise, for a full course of treatment, six to eight sessions at weekly intervals. In China, the treatment sessions are often repeated at more frequent intervals, but this does not seem to be necessary, especially for the more chronic conditions. The results certainly seem to be as good (see Chapter 8).

Generally, if treatment is successful, the effects will last six months or more. In self-limiting conditions, complete resolution is not uncommon. It is perfectly feasible to have, say, six-monthly 'top-up' treatments in the more chronic conditions.

After the first treatment, one of three things will happen: no change, worsening of symptoms (syn. *aggravation* in homeopathy) or improvement, sometimes amounting to complete resolution. The latter frequently occurs in the more acute conditions and it may be that no more treatment is necessary. In the more chronic conditions, there may be no improvement for several sessions – if there is no improvement after the third treatment, it is generally best to admit failure and give up. This is only true provided that the proper points have been properly treated – it may pay to think again and look, not only at your point selection, but also your technique. If there is aggravation, it is very likely that the acupuncture will work. It is obviously important to familiarize the patient with the possible changes in their symptomatology – otherwise you will end up with a significant drop-out rate! With more persistent aggravation or with high reactors, it is often advisable to decrease the amount of stimulation in subsequent treatments.

SAFETY

With certain provisos, and in the right hands, acupuncture is safe, this being one of its major attractions.

A certain amount of anatomical knowledge is essential. At the very least, one ought to know what lies beneath the channel markings! With this knowledge and the guidelines given in this chapter, there ought to be no problem.

Probably the easiest mistake is to puncture the pleura with the risk of pneumothorax. This will be avoided if one-inch needles are *not* inserted to their hilts on the chest wall – special care is needed with G.B.21 and points around that area (see 'Specific Points'). Entering large blood vessels does not seem to pose a problem. This is common in say U.B.40, but, perhaps due to the fineness of the needles, bleeding of any significance is rare. The avoidance of bruising or haematoma was discussed earlier.

With the increasing problem of AIDS, needle sterility is of the utmost importance. Certainly AIDS and hepatitis B pose the greatest threat of spread of serious infection. It has been shown[5] that immersion of the needles in an antiseptic solution is *not* sufficient. The minimum requirement is *proper autoclaving* but disposable needles are the ideal. Despite their expense, I would advocate their use exclusively. I would further recommend, for the operator's safety, that protective gloves are worn if there is even the most minor open wound on the operator's hands. By the same token, take extreme care when handling the needles. As in conventional medicine, it is mandatory to dispose of your needles (disposable and 'finished' re-usables) after use into a 'cin-bin' for incineration. Provided a normal standard of hygiene is observed, minor soft tissue infection is very unusual. Occasionally, a small urticarial wheal is produced at the puncture site but it usually disappears quickly and is of little consequence.

5
SPECIFIC CONDITIONS

I will now go through some of the more common conditions amenable to acupuncture treatment and enumerate the respective commonly used points. Most of this chapter will be based on treatment using the 'local and distal point' method as I believe that, not only is it a good way to start, but, for many, is a continually successful method of treating musculoskeletal conditions. Purists will argue that treating these conditions on a local level, without considering the systemic factors, gives poor results because the treatment is so superficial. I think this is nonsense and it is certainly not borne out in the results (Chapter 8). However, this is not to say that systemic factors are not important. They may well play a part in the pathogenesis of musculoskeletal disease and due reference to this will be given in the next chapter. My point is that you will still get good results using the local methods, and, as these are comparatively much easier to learn and comprehend, these will form the rationale behind the treatment of the following conditions. My only exceptions in this chapter are the last two conditions described – migraine and neuralgias. I have included two systemic points, based purely and empirically on traditional teaching. It is not unreasonable to suppose that migraine may be caused by something more than just local dysfunction of channels, and after all – the whole of acupuncture is empirical!

LOW BACK PAIN (AND SCIATICA)

This probably accounts for the largest group seeking acupuncture and it is not difficult to see why. Our surgeries are full of such cases – a large proportion of these are understandably disillusioned with conventional medicine, whose results are not outstanding in that department.

The diagnoses include a multitude of conditions: disc syndromes, muscular strain, osteoarthroses, ankylosing spondylitis, to mention but a few. A large proportion do not fit into any conventional diagnostic category at all. For our purposes this is unimportant – the methodology will be similar. Most of these patients would have been through the conventional diagnostic and treatment procedures and are seeking a trial of acupuncture because of unsatisfactory results or an unwillingness to take potentially dangerous drugs. It is assumed that potentially treatable diseases (conventionally) have been excluded first (neoplasia, osteomalacia, renal disease, Paget's disease, osteoporosis, severe or persistent disc prolapse etc.), and that general and specific conventional measures of proven benefit (e.g. weight loss in obesity) have or are being applied.

LOCAL POINTS

For the detection of *Ashi* and treatment, the patient has to be lying face down, flat. One or more *ashi* will usually be found along the U.B. **Channels**, but there may well be others, not on a definite channel. Patients will frequently pinpoint centres of pain and these can also be treated as *ashi*, even if not tender (though they often will be). Sometimes, quite firm pressure will be needed to elicit the *ashi*. If pain is felt or radiated into the buttock areas, the important **Key point** is G.B. 30. This is also mandatory for sciatica and is thought to be the most important point in that condition.

DISTAL POINTS

Invariably U.B.40. If there is radiation of pain down the lateral aspect of the leg, G.B.34 must be used; also G.B.40 if radiation extends to the foot.

SHOULDER/NECK DISORDERS

I make no apology for including these all together as, despite the differing pathologies, the acupuncture treatment will often be similar and involve the same channels and key points.

The main neck pathologies are cervical disc lesions and cervical spondylosis. In the shoulder, there are the various rotator cuff syndromes (subacromial bursitis, supraspinatus tendinitis, etc.), capsulitis, strains and arthritis. Again, it is important not to get too bogged down with precise diagnoses; often there is a mixture of conventional pathologies present, with secondary soft tissue trigger points. The all-important thing is to find the *ashi*. The same provisos apply to this section as in low back pain.

LOCAL POINTS

The patient is best treated sitting up, but back supported, on a couch. In the neck the *Ashi* will be found most frequently along the U.B. and G.B. channels, to one or both sides of the midline. For the detection of other *ashi*, it is important to palpate the whole area between the cervical spine and the deltoid. Posteriorly, *ashi* often lie along the S.I. channel and on the G.B. channel between G.B.20 and G.B.21. Superiorly and laterally, the L.I. and S.J. channels are often involved. Again, I stress that *ashi* do not have to lie exactly on channels – it is far more important to find the tender points wherever they are. When dealing with the more specific soft tissue rheumatisms, the *ashi* will be found in their conventional places. Where you would put in your needle for steroid injection, put in an acupuncture needle (including the joints) – this statement really applies to all the conditions.

Two very important **Key points** are G.B.20 and G.B.21. I would use these in all shoulder/neck disorders. In shoulder pain, use L.I.14 and L.I.15.

DISTAL POINTS

According to channel involvement, the most useful will be L.I.11, L.I.4, S.I.3, S.J.5, U.B.60 and G.B.34. S.J.5 is especially useful for pain and radiation on the lateral aspect of the upper limb which is not on a clearly defined channel.

TENNIS ELBOW

LOCAL POINTS

One looks for the main *Ashi* exactly as if for a conventional local steroid injection. This will usually be found over the lateral epicondyle and is often pin-pointed by the patient. The pain and tenderness can be easily reproduced on forced internal rotation of the forearm or by picking up a heavyish object with the forearm pronated. Sometimes there will be other *ashi*, either in the vicinity of the epicondyle or further away, particularly down the L.I. channel. It is important that all *ashi* are searched for and treated. It will be found helpful to insert the needles obliquely. There is a fallacy that for injection to be successful, it has to hurt – this is invariably due to putting the needle right through the tendon or beyond! Oblique insertion will make it easier to end up just puncturing the tendon sheath and nothing else. The production of the right type of *deqi* (which should *not* be horrendously painful) will confirm the correct location.

The **Key local point** is L.I.11.

DISTAL POINTS

Careful siting of the pain of radiation is necessary. The more medial it is, the more likely that L.I.4 will be used; more laterally, S.J.5. If in doubt, use S.J.5.

GOLFER'S ELBOW

LOCAL POINTS

Use any *Ashi* as per tennis elbow – invariably around the medial epicondyle.

DISTAL POINTS

H.7 – if the pain is radiated along that channel – if not, distal point not necessary.

TENOSYNOVITIS (AND CARPAL TUNNEL SYNDROME)

This condition can occur in any tendon but more commonly in the forearm, wrist and hand. Merely treat the *Ashi* without any key or distal points. As per conventional medicine, the needle point must end up in the tendon sheath, *not* in the tendon. Oblique insertion will make life easier.

ARTHRITIS WRIST

All types of arthritis can produce trouble at this joint. Careful palpation around all aspects of the point will elicit *Ashi* and these should all be treated. A lot of these points will go into the joint but do not be frightened by this prospect – as I have said previously, side effects, including infection, are rare. Distal points are not necessary.

HIP DISORDERS

A lot of these will have osteoarthrosis or other forms of arthritis. Pain can be centred in the hip in sacroiliitis and sciatica; various soft tissue rheumatisms occur around the hip, including trochanteric bursitis.

LOCAL POINTS

From a practical point of view, one has to decide whether to treat anteriorly or posteriorly, or one following the other, as there will often be local points on both aspects. Start by getting the patient to identify the main seat (so to speak) of the pain which will commonly be on one aspect. *Ashi*, which can be anywhere around the joint, are then searched for. If there is any doubt, turn the patient over and examine the other aspect for *ashi*. The *ashi* will more frequently be found along the channels of radiated pain: U.B. posteriorly, G.B. laterally and St. anteriorly.

The important **Key points** are G.B.29 and St.31. *G.B.30 is used for any pain felt posteriorly.*

DISTAL POINTS

The site(s) of maximal pain or radiation is the key factor – U.B.40 for pain felt along the posterior aspect of the thigh, G.B.34 lateral aspect, and St.36 (or St.44) anterior aspect.

KNEE DISORDERS

Probably the commonest disorder is osteoarthrosis. Slow-to-resolve sprains and soft tissue rheumatisms, such as bursitis, are also amenable to acupuncture. Once again, it is assumed that conventionally correctable conditions, such as medial meniscus lesions and gout, are excluded.

LOCAL POINTS

Ashi can be found on any aspect of the joint. The main **Key points** to use are St.35, Sp.9 and U.B.40. From the practical point of view, using all three key points will often necessitate two 'sittings' as St.35 and Sp.9 are best approached with the leg supine and U.B.40 is approached posteriorly. If there is a time constraint, I would opt for St.35 and Sp.9. However, it is sometimes possible to insert the above two needles with the leg supine and then carefully turn the patient over and insert U.B.40.

DISTAL POINTS

Not necessary, unless there is clearly defined radiated pain; then use St.36 and/or St.44 for anterior pain, U.B.60 for posterior pain, and G.B.34 and/or G.B.40 for lateral pain. For pain radiated down the medial aspect of the leg (unusual), consult Chapter 3 for correct channel identification and then treat the appropriate distal point: Sp.6, Liv.3 or K.3.

NEURALGIAS

I am including in this section the classical (trigeminal) and atypical facial neuralgias, and herpes zoster. Like migraine, these must represent something more than just local channel dysfunction. As well as applying local and distal point theory, I am also including a systemic point for the first time. The brief of this chapter is to describe the commonly used points for certain conditions so I will attempt not to stray from this. Chapter 6 will give a very basic resumé of systemic theory, but, for the purposes of this book, the use of these points must be seen to be entirely empirical.

LOCAL POINTS

It is important in neuralgias not to needle within the neuralgic area. This seems to go against the grain of our usual method but needling these areas very often *worsens* the condition. Use **Circumferential points** by 'ringing' the painful area (or lesions in herpes zoster) with three or four randomly inserted needles. Some acupuncturists treat *ashi* on the opposite side ('mirror points') but I have no experience of this.

DISTAL POINTS

These are deduced in the usual way by carefully mapping the area of pain and radiation and treating the distal points of the relevant channels. Generally speaking, in facial pain, G.B.34 or G.B.40 will cover the lateral aspect of the face, St.44 more anteriorly, L.I.4 the lower jaw area, and

U.B.60 more medially sited pain. If in doubt, treat all these points (consult Chapter 3). The same principles of distal point selection will apply to herpes zoster. Virtually any channel can be affected here.

Treat **Systemic point Liv.3, Bilaterally.** As a general rule, when using systemic points, treat both sides.

MIGRAINE

I am including migraine in this chapter as it seems to fall into the same broad category of chronic/recurrent painful conditions not always successfully treated by conventional means. What is more, there is a similar response rate to acupuncture as in musculoskeletal conditions.

Apart from classical migraine, I would also include any chronic/recurring headaches, with the usual proviso that potentially serious diseases have been excluded. Cluster migraines seem to respond particularly well.

Although one could treat the acute attacks, this treatment is more recommended as a full course to serve as a prophylactic. The beneficial effects will often last six months or more, and, as with the previous conditions, 'top-ups' can be given in the course of time.

LOCAL POINTS

Most patients with migraine and chronic tension headaches will have *Ashi* in the scalp. Many sufferers will be able to accurately pinpoint these, especially during or soon after an attack. They are often palpable as little nodules and they are vital to treat. In most generalized or hemicranial headaches, I would include the following **Key local points**: G.B.20, G.B.19, G.B.14, G.B.8, and **Extra point temple** (one cun posterior to midpoint between lateral end of eyebrow and outer acanthus). These, as the *ashi*, would be used on both sides with bilateral headaches, or the one side in purely unilateral headaches. Occasionally, very localized headaches can be treated with the relevant local points (for example, G.B.19 and G.B.20 in occipital headaches (where I usually add in G.B.21)) but one usually ends up finding *ashi* all over the place!

DISTAL POINTS

Use U.B.60, and G.B.34 *or* G.B.40, on one or both sides, as in local points. Treat **Systemic points**, Sp.6 and Liv.3, on both sides.

6
SYSTEMIC TREATMENT

Firstly, let us get this chapter in perspective. The main purpose of this book is to present a method of acupuncture treatment suitable for conventional practising clinicians, such as has been outlined in the preceding chapters. The factors governing the choice of this method include – simplicity, ease of learning, effectiveness and logistical practicality. It can form a useful part of a therapeutic armamentarium in a conventional setting.

It has to be realised that this method is but a very small part of an enormous subject. To present to you a total treatise of acupuncture would, I am sure, put many of you off and leave you little wiser (and myself with an awesome brief).

The purist traditionalist would argue that it is necessary to understand, learn and apply, the whole of traditional Chinese medicine before treating patients; that even musculoskeletal conditions involve systemic disturbances. One would certainly not argue with this principle, which counters 'treating the symptoms, not the cause'. However, in practice, this view is just *not* substantiated. Treatment on a local level, as I have described it, *is* effective for these conditions. This is just as well, as, otherwise, I doubt many of us would be practising any form of acupuncture!

The purpose of this chapter (and indeed Chapter 7) is to give you a brief outline of all the other ideas that go to make up the discipline of traditional Chinese acupuncture. More perspective can be gained, bearing in mind that the 'local' methods are a very small part of what is a highly ordered and rational system that has its roots in ancient Chinese philosophy. One owes a certain respect to a system that may well, in time, be found to produce acceptable medical results, despite the present unacceptability of many of its principles. We have to study these principles in order to be able to make any sense of the rationale behind traditional Chinese medicine as a whole. Only then may we eventually be in a position to find a scientific basis for acupuncture.

From a more practical point of view, there may be many of you who wish to treat patients from a broader base, especially those with the more chronic diseases/symptom complexes who have not responded to conventional medicine. Although the subject matter will be dealt with relatively superficially, there may be enough information to enable you to work out a trial of treatment. Anyone willing and interested in these wider aspects of acupuncture should, however, consider further study as coverage here can only be brief.

YIN–YANG

This is a philosophical concept of two opposing but interdependent forces that are constantly changing but maintain a total equilibrium in health. Yang is more positive, active and hot – Yin is negative, hypoactive and cold. Each organ has an element of Yin and Yang in it – with a preponderance of one. The liver for example is mainly Yang and the kidney mainly Yin.

Disease occurs when Yin and Yang no longer balance, either because one is in excess (a *'Shi'* disease – commonly acute) or deficient (a *'Xu'* disease – commonly chronic). The aim of traditional Chinese diagnosis is to find the organ(s) that is causing the imbalance and any pathogen that may be harming that organ, and then to treat the organ(s) and pathogenic invasion by acupuncture.

The vital energy, or *qi* (Chapter 1), that supplies the organs flows along the corresponding channels. It is the correction of the flow of qi along these channels that forms the basis of acupuncture treatment of organ dysfunction. This correction will rectify the Yin–Yang balance of that organ, and therefore of the body, provided the pathogens are treated as well. Various acupuncture points (and methods) are described (see later) that help to dispel pathogenic invasion – these must be similarly treated.

In brief: find the dysfunctioning organ(s), identify the pathogens (if any) and treat the corresponding points.

ORGANS

The following revision will remind us that the functions of the organs in traditional Chinese medicine are often quite different from their conventional equivalents:

Heart: Dominates the circulation of blood. Keeps the mind healthy.

Liver: Maintains the free flow of blood and *qi* through the body.

Spleen: Governs digestion and blood. Maintains muscle bulk.

Lung: Controls respiration and the passage of 'water'. Dominates the hair and skin.

Kidney: Dominates growth and reproduction. Produces marrow. Controls body water.

Pericardium: As in conventional medicine.

Sanjiao: Otherwise known as 'the three cavities' or the 'triple warmer organ', no apparent conventional equivalent, seems to encompass areas in the chest, epigastrium, and hypogastrium – functionally controls body temperature.

The following organs seem to have similar functions to their conventional equivalents: **Small intestine, gall bladder, stomach, large intestine, urinary bladder.**

We can apply some of this teaching in attempting to identify organ dysfunction (in traditional Chinese terms) in our patients. For instance, knowing that the spleen is the main organ that governs digestion, would make the spleen the main target organ to treat in digestive disorders (e.g. irritable bowel syndrome). Apart from this knowledge, there are traditional signs described (see later) which attempt to pinpoint organ dysfunction more accurately. It has to be admitted, however, that a lot of the 'organ points' that are described in traditional teaching seem to be chosen very empirically, no doubt born out of long experience (e.g. liver and spleen in migraine). There are a whole host of points described that are suitable for various symptoms and symptom complexes – beyond the scope of this book to list completely but worthy of further study if you are interested in practising 'systemic' acupuncture.

ORGAN TREATMENT

There is a lot of theory here, which is not totally agreed upon. I have taken the simplistic view that if you treat the distal point on that channel (as described in Chapter 3), you will treat that organ. The traditionalists will shudder in horror at this gross oversimplification but it does have the merit of being easier to learn! I will, however, describe some of the ideas in traditional teaching.

The first principle is that a diseased organ will need either 'tonifying' or 'sedating'. Generally, with a *Xu* disease the organ will need tonifying, with a *Shi* disease, sedating. There are five 'elements' described in Chinese philosophy: wood, fire, earth, metal and water, each having a creating or destroying relationship with another (e.g. wood creates fire, fire creates earth, water destroys fire). The creator element is called the 'mother' element and the created element the 'son' element. Each organ is represented by an element (e.g. heart – fire) and the mother element to that organ is used to tonify that organ, the son element, to sedate. Each organ has five *'shu'* points described, each representing one of the elements. You will be relieved to hear that I am not about to list these points!

I suspect that my simplistic choice of distal points relies heavily on the supposition that the majority of diseases affecting a particular organ will be either *Xu* or *Shi*. Hence the use of one distal point per organ will cover most eventualities. For example H.7 is the earth *shu* point for the heart (the son to fire) and most diseases of the heart are *Shi* in nature.

CHANNEL LINKS

In traditional textbooks, many interconnecting links between channels are described. These have an obvious practical advantage, i.e. one point will often serve to treat several others. Some of these links will be described.

The *'luo'* connecting points are those connecting one channel with another. To give you an idea, I have listed the organs and the channels to which they are linked in Table 3. I have omitted the points themselves as they are not relevant to learn at this stage.

Yet more points that represent the surface points of the organs are described – the *'mu'* points are on the front and the 'shu' points are on the back. The *shu* points are more effective for the Yin organs, and the *mu* points for the Yang organs. Again, these will not be listed here.

PATHOGENS

The traditional Chinese pathogens have already been listed: heat, cold, wind, damp and phlegm. These are believed to be secondary invaders in that the primary pathology is in the Yin–Yang imbalance; this allows the invasion of pathogens which have to be treated as well to ensure successful therapy.

Table 3 Linked channels

Organ /Channel	Linked channel
Liver	Gall bladder
Kidney	Urinary bladder
Heart	Small intestine
Lung	Large intestine
Spleen	Stomach
Pericardium	*Sanjiao*

HEAT

This is usually equivalent to infection or febrile illness, usually acute, but also is involved with any condition producing 'warmth' (gout, phlebitis, acute trauma). The points to disperse heat are L.I.4 and L.I.11.

COLD

Invasion of cold usually occurs in more chronic diseases, especially the longstanding soft tissue rheumatisms (e.g. frozen shoulder). This is not terribly unconventional as physiotherapists will often treat these conditions with heat (and the above with cold applications). In China, the burning of *'Moxa'* is used (dried *Artemesis vulgaris* plant), either actually on a needle to heat it up, or in the form of a 'stick' which is held close to the point. The *ashi* are the main points to treat with heat. *Moxa* sticks can be purchased in this country (Chapter 9) and have the advantage of supplying very localized heat which is traditionally regarded as fundamentally important. Apparently, diffuse heat will not give the same result.

The main disadvantage of *moxa* sticks is that the fumes stink! More modern forms of local heat include rather expensive infra-red devices.

WIND

Invasion of wind occurs in many diseases, characterized by changeability of symptoms, not only in character, but also in site. As with the above pathogens, patients affected thus will often complain of their dislike of that pathogen or that their symptoms are made worse by the same. Examples include various allergic conditions and arthralgias.

Points to disperse wind are L.I.4. and L.I.11.

DAMP

This is more difficult to define. Conditions where damp invades are often described as having the following characteristics: greasiness, stickiness, stagnancy, 'heavy' feeling. These are to us very conceptual terms but examples include chronic weepy skin diseases, obesity and acne. Damp will more often than not invade via a dysfunctioning spleen so the traditional signs (see later) are similar.

The point to disperse damp is St.40 (midway between the tip of the lateral malleolus and the lateral knee joint line – one- or one-and-a-half-inch needle – perpendicular direction).

PHLEGM

This is a true secondary invader and occurs, not only in the form of its conventional equivalent (e.g. chronic bronchitis), but also in chronic suppuration, catarrhal conditions, ascites and strokes. Damp and phlegm often co-exist, and both are more likely to enter with a dysfunctioning spleen – hence the common additional use of Sp.6 when the above two pathogens are involved.

The point to disperse phlegm is St.40 (see above).

TRADITIONAL CHINESE DIAGNOSTIC SIGNS

Using our skills and knowledge of conventional medicine, and applying them to the aforementioned concepts, we would, surprisingly often, be able to form some sort of diagnosis in traditional Chinese medical terms – which may form the rationale behind a plan of acupuncture treatment. There exist, however, special signs that are taught in traditional Chinese medicine to aid more specific diagnosis. Some of these signs are completely unconventional and so will be difficult for us to learn, let alone give credibility to. As with the rest of this book, a completely open mind is necessary for this forms part of basic teaching and hence should be studied with a like mind. I will confine myself to the signs unfamiliar to us – many other signs are described but these are more or less as in conventional medicine.

TONGUE

Two parts of the tongue are described: the 'tongue proper' is the red rim around the edge of the tongue – normally pale red; the 'tongue coating' is the normally thin, whitish coating on top of the tongue.

A red tongue proper can be caused by liver disease or a chronic disease of heat; a more purplish-red colour can indicate a more acute disease of heat; while a purplish colour indicates heart disease. A pale tooth-marked tongue proper can be due to kidney or spleen dysfunction.

A white greasy tongue coating indicates invasion of damp and/or phlegm, and usually spleen disease too. An opaque white coating can mean invasion of cold, and a yellow coating, of heat (and smoking!). A deficient tongue coating can indicate kidney disease or marked deficiency of *Yin*.

PULSE

In classical Chinese medicine, there are six pulses described at each wrist. These comprise three positions on the radial artery, each having a deep and superficial pulse. Each pulse is supposed to represent an organ. I feel it would take so long to become skilled and familiar with this system that further description would be pointless.

However, a slightly easier form of pulse diagnosis, called 'pulse generalization', is also used. This is still difficult for us to comprehend and elicit, but, like tongue diagnosis, it may be worthy of practice.

A *Xu* pulse is described as weak or thready and disappears on heavy pressure. By definition, this is seen in chronic diseases of Yin–Yang deficiency and often indicates splenic dysfunction. A *Shi* pulse is the opposite, forceful, and obviously seen in *Shi* diseases. A 'bowstring' pulse is harder and more forceful but more flexible like a bowstring and can indicate liver dysfunction.

I certainly would not trust myself to elicit any of these pulse changes with confidence but will continue to practice! Many other pulse generalizations are taught, mostly equivalent to conventional pulse abnormalities.

What is fascinating when reading about these unconventional ideas is that they are immersed in a mass of very conventional and plausible medical principles. One is left with the feeling that "they can't have made it up", and "is it us that have just missed observing these signs and so discounted them?". One could apply this thought process to many parts, if not the whole, of this book!

SUMMARY

To make a choice of acupuncture points for a given patient, when applying classical Chinese medical principles, one looks at three areas:

(1)   Local dysfunction of channels

(2)   Organ dysfunction

(3)   Pathogen invasion

In the preceding chapters, we have dealt with (1) in detail, together with the use and selection of local and distal points. Indeed the main scope of this book is to advocate this technique as the best introduction to acupuncture, and, for some, the only technique. In keeping with this chapter, however, we have taken one step beyond! Certainly there will be conditions in Chapter 5 that may have organ dysfunction and pathogen invasion, and it may be worthwhile seeking and treating these if local methods are not successful.

In any painful 'systemic disease', local and distal points are used in exactly the same way. Migraine has already been discussed but irritable bowel, sinusitis and more chronic painful conditions should have their local channel dysfunction sought and treated.

By comparison, we have only been able to look at (2) and (3) briefly in this chapter. Using some of the pointers described and our knowledge of conventional medicine, there will be occasions, however, when it will be possible to form an opinion of likely organ dysfunction and pathogen involvement. Various examples will be given below, but remember, above all, that you are not likely to do any harm if you get it wrong! Many of these conditions are inadequately treated conventionally and your patients will be only too grateful for you to try something else on these occasions.

EXAMPLES

These are all conditions and symptom complexes that are familiar enough to all of us. Therefore it goes without saying that all necessary conventional precautions have been taken before embarking on acupuncture treatment, either therapeutically or by investigation.

Although based on traditional teaching, my guidelines can only be brief in a book of this type. Due credit cannot really be given to the complex thinking behind the various prescriptions, but a lot of it is fairly dogmatic and empirical in any case. Always look for organ dysfunction and pathogen invasion, not necessarily described in these prescriptions – if you find them treat them; for many of the more chronic diseases have multiple interrelated organ pathologies. To discuss all these possibilities is well beyond the scope of this book (and its author). Remember when using systemic points (organ and pathogens) to treat *both* sides.

ARTHRITIS

Local and distal points must be treated, as described previously.

The other important entity is pathogen invasion. In the more chronic forms of arthritis, cold and damp are said to invade. Therefore the additional point to use will be St.40. Heat should be used on the *ashi*. In more acute arthritis, heat will be the pathogen so L.I.4 should be used. In 'flitting' or 'wandering' arthritis, wind is often involved – L.I.4 or L.I.11 should then be treated.

LOW BACK PAIN

In recurrent back pain, which is often worse in the cold and damp, there may be pathogen invasion of damp, wind and cold. In this case, in addition to local and distal points, add L.I.4 (or L.I.11), St.40 and local heat. The same logic can be applied to sciatica.

FROZEN SHOULDER

In the early stages, wind and damp invade – later, cold. Therefore, in addition to local and distal points, treat St.40, L.I.4 or L.I.11, and local heat.

OTHER SOFT TISSUE RHEUMATISM

Likely pathogens are wind and cold — therefore use local and distal points, heat and L.I.4.

DEPRESSION

This is believed to occur because of *Xu* of the heart, spleen and kidney. The points to treat are P.6, H.7, Sp.6, K.3 and St.36. (St.36 is often described as a general tonifier and regulator of the stomach.)

ANXIETY

Anxiety and depression very often coexist, but anxiety taken on its own is believed to be caused by hyperactivity of Yang of the liver. 'Tension' headaches, irritability and anger are more prominent in this entity and the points should include Liv.3 and L.I.4.

VERTIGO AND TINNITUS

These symptoms are often due to pathology about which nothing much can be done, conventionally. In Chinese medicine, the pathogens involved are phlegm and damp, and the organs, spleen and kidney. The points used are St.40, Sp.6, K.3, H.7 and P.6.The last two are 'symptomatic' points.

DYSPEPSIA

It is assumed, of course, that conventional investigation and treatment have been applied. The main organs dysfunctioning are the spleen, liver and stomach. The points to treat are Sp.6, Liv.3 and St.36. In addition, P.6 can be used (symptomatic for nausea).

IRRITABLE BOWEL SYNDROME

This is another example where it is useful to treat the local channel dysfunction as well as the systemic disturbance. Use the **Distal points** of the site of pain, as well as the following systemic points: Sp.6, St.36 and L.I.4.

CHRONIC BRONCHITIS

As we all know, alleviation of symptoms is all we can hope to achieve here. Wind, phlegm and cold (or heat in acute infective exacerbations) are all involved pathogens. Apart from the lungs, the following organs are usually involved: kidney, spleen and liver. The points will include Lu.7, L.I.11, St.40, K.3, Sp.6 and Liv.3.

ASTHMA

Again, wind, phlegm and heat (or cold) are the likely pathogens. The organ dysfunction is mainly lung, spleen and kidney. A typical prescription would be: Lu.7, St.40, L.I.11, Sp.6 and K.3.Various points on the *Ren* channel are described which are supposed to aid bronchodilatation but I have no experience of these.

SINUSITIS

Use local and distal points referable to the pain and tenderness. Not surprisingly, wind, phlegm and cold (heat in acute attacks) are the pathogens. The main organ dysfunction in chronic sinusitis is a *qi* deficiency in the lungs. Additional points are St.40, L.I.4 (and/or L.I.11) and Lu.7.

MENOPAUSAL FLUSHES

The points used here are really symptomatic: Liv.3 and P.6.

NAUSEA (INCLUDING PREGNANCY NAUSEA AND SICKNESS)

This is only mentioned due to the current (understandable) aversion to taking drugs during pregnancy. The stomach and spleen are the organs involved; in addition the symptomatic point for nausea is used: St.36, Sp.6 and P.6.

7
OTHER FORMS OF ACUPUNCTURE

The form of acupuncture demonstrated in this book is the basic classical method – certainly the oldest and still the most popularly practised form. The principles comprise selection of acupuncture points on the twenty-six body channels, inserting needles into these points, and manually manipulating them.

Other forms of acupuncture exist which either use sites other than the classical channels, or that differ in the method of point treatment and/or 'stimulation'. It is not the brief of this book to describe these in any detail as they go well beyond the introductory stage; many of them are comparatively modern. However, using the logic of the previous chapter, there may be occasions when you will be interested in trying one of these forms albeit in a rather superficial way; or you may be stimulated to study further. More details will be given to those areas that you could attempt to practise and obtain good results.

ELECTRO-ACUPUNCTURE

This is using electrical impulses to 'stimulate' an acupuncture needle. Its main uses are in acupuncture anaesthesia (Chapter 8) but it can also be used in 'normal' acupuncture. It offers a more scientifically controlled method of point stimulation/treatment, but the science behind its use is, to say the least, vague and ill understood.   Let me say here and now that manual stimulation is still regarded as effective in the methods that have been described and that electrical methods offer little advantage.   However, it is widely used and so its methodology will be discussed.

The machines used are specialized, as they conform to a fairly strict standard. A pulsed, direct current is used, with a square wave form (a sine wave would burn the flesh). Not only is the amplitude accurately controllable, but also the frequency.

Another alterable parameter is the use of 'interrupted' waves (recurring periods of absence of impulses) which is supposed to stop adaptation to the stimulus. Yet another variation is 'modulation' when there is one main frequency, modulated by a higher frequency wave, perhaps at specific intervals. There is not yet enough known to be able to comment on these variants, so we will stick to the straight forward principles.

Each output from the machine ends in two electrodes – one black coloured (negative), the other red (positive). It follows that for current to flow, **both** electrodes must be connected to the patient. The connections are usually crocodile clips, attachable to the handles (metallic only – see Chapter 4) of the acupuncture needles. If only one needle is required for treatment, the other electrode can be, for example, held in the hand of the patient (perhaps by connection to a hand-held electrode which is made for that purpose). Better machines have several outputs with the obvious potential of treating more points at a time.

It is paramount before connecting up, that proper point location and *deqi* have been accomplished using manual techniques. The machine is switched on with the amplitude adjusters turned right down. The frequency is adjusted first. From experience, it has been found that the optimum frequency for pain relief is 5 Hz or less. The more modern machines, using digital technology, can adjust the frequency very accurately indeed. Much work is needed in the future to find out more about which frequencies are best for particular purposes. The above guideline is without scientific basis but is the best we can do at the moment!

Next the amplitude of the relevant output(s) is turned up slowly until the patient feels a not unpleasant 'tingly' sensation. This is usually felt in one electrode – more often, but not always, in the negative one. Apparently, it is not important which point receives the most sensation, but I, quite empirically, prefer the *ashi* to get the stimulus. If this is not the case, I simply swap the electrodes around. The patient will adapt to the stimulus and the amplitude can be slowly turned up again, perhaps by the patient, until the stimulus is felt again. This can be done recurrently each time adaptation occurs. Sometimes muscle twitching occurs in response to the electrical stimulation – this need not cause concern, but, if of sufficient violence, could conceivably cause needle breakage. **Slow** turning up of the amplitude should avoid this.

Most sessions will last 10–30 minutes. Before switching off the machine, it is vital that the **electrodes are disconnected first;** otherwise 'kick-back' can occur, causing a nasty shock.

The main advantage of electro-acupuncture that I see is the ability to use mild, prolonged, controllable stimulation. This may have its attributes, especially in a first treatment, but, as stated before, is no replacement for correct manual technique. Among the obvious disadvantages are expense and time consumption. The main contra-indication to the use of electro-acupuncture is the presence of a pacemaker but the passing of currents across the chest should be avoided in anyone with a history of heart disease.

There is a present vogue for using electrical therapy without needles – by simply using a probe on an acupuncture point. Much evaluation has yet to be done before one can comment on whether or not this is effective.

This method is distinct from transcutaneous nerve stimulation (TNS) which has been widely used for some time. Here, similar sorts of currents are used, but each electrode is in the form of a flat piece of rubber, held in place on the patient's skin at strategic areas, usually corresponding to the sites of maximal pain and/or tenderness. The 'stimulation' is obviously more diffuse and comparatively little knowledge is needed for its use.

Many of the studies cited in Chapter 8 relate to TNS as well as acupuncture. It almost certainly works in the same way as acupuncture and studies have indicated[6,7] that it is probably as effective in pain relief. The major advantage is that it can be used by inadequately qualified personnel, including the patients themselves – small, portable TNS machines are made especially for this purpose. From a practitioner's point of view, the disadvantage is the time element – the treatment sessions take longer and have to be performed more frequently.

Another more modern dimension to acupuncture and electronics comes under the banner of 'Bio-electronic Regulatory Medicine'. This is comparatively modern, and indeed so distinct that it is completely beyond the scope of this book. This discipline explores the possibility of detecting electrical changes at certain body points, reflecting dysfunction of particular organs, and then correcting the dysfunction by means of acupuncture or homeopathic medicines. The theory relies heavily on the notion that the homeopathic remedies have demonstrable electrical properties that can even aid in the 'electrical diagnostic' process. I would recommend that you only regard this branch with open interest at the moment (see Chapter 8).

EAR ACUPUNCTURE

This must be regarded as relatively modern as the French were the first to invent it (still hotly debated!). There are many facets to ear acupuncture – some very modern and advanced. To simplify matters, I will deal only with the more straightforward facets that form a useful background to this immense sub-speciality. This limited information will, however, lend itself to the possibility of the reader being able to practice some basic auricular therapy. There are a number of more advanced and highly comprehensive techniques of ear acupuncture that need a textbook in themselves! These will not be discussed here.

Ear acupuncture is based on the theory that over the ear are situated acupuncture points which correspond to various parts of the body – somatic and visceral. This is distinct to the channels and points previously described. Figure 17 shows a selection of these points over the anterior surface of the ear:

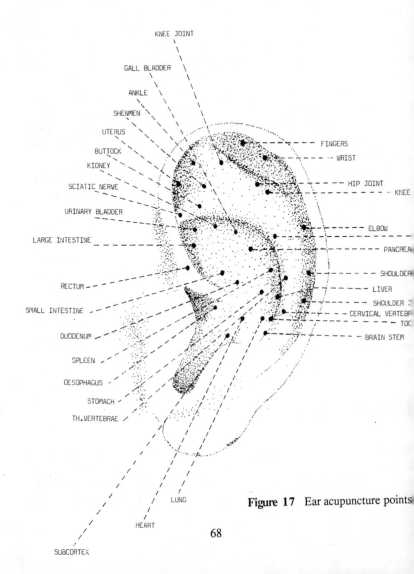

Figure 17 Ear acupuncture points

A lot of this book has probably produced a healthy degree of scepticism but this will take the prize! And yet ear acupuncture forms a vital basis to probably the greatest demonstration of the efficacy of acupuncture: **anaesthesia** (Chapter 8). On a smaller scale, we will explore a simple technique of pain relief using ear acupuncture.

Just as one searches for *ashis* in the traditional way, one looks for the 'sensitive point' on the ear. This will usually corrrespond to the appropriate area shown in Figure 17. In a patient with any pain (especially acute pain), such a sensitive point will be found and *this* is the point to be treated. The method of locating this point is important. One uses some sort of probe, e.g. the closed end of a ballpoint pen or some such implement. There are purpose-built, spring-loaded devices available. The vital thing is to apply firm and equal pressure when probing an area. (An idea of the area can be gleaned by consulting Figure 17.) There will always, eventually, be found one single point which is more painful than any other – this is the sensitive point.

The point is treated by inserting a half-inch needle obliquely into (not through!) the ear. Manipulation is accomplished by rotatory means only (no up-and-down movement), and, if *deqi* is experienced, it will be comparatively painful. However, the reward will be amply demonstrated, as, in the case of acute pain, there will be immediate relief!

This is the ideal way for sceptics to try ear acupuncture as it is so simple and gives immediate feedback.

The problem with this method is the limited duration of analgesia. In order to produce more long-term effects, 'semi-permanent' needles can be inserted, remaining in place for 1–3 weeks. There are various types available but I would recommend the newer disposable ones (for the same reasons as in Chapter 4). There are left *in situ* and 'stimulated' by the patient whenever analgesia is required.

On a wider scale, one can treat the 'organ' points either using the principles of traditional Chinese medicine, as already discussed, or applying conventional principles with regard to known organ or somatic pathology. However, the 'treatment' of such points is kept standard in that there is one point per structure and this point is used whatever the nature of the dysfunction, being treated in exactly the same way as described in the previous paragraphs. Use the ear point(s) on the affected side in unilateral conditions; on the dominant side in bilateral or 'systemic' conditions. You will notice one point which is not structure-related: *shenmen*. This is described as a sedative point and is apparently useful as a general anxiolytic.

Ear acupuncture treatment for tobacco addiction and weight reduction is very popular but, in my opinion, not of great benefit. Unfortunately these conditions lend themselves to this sort of practice – the patients are desperate, and conventional approaches are not brimming with success. The 'theory' behind the selection of appropriate points is questionable: the stomach point for dieting, the lung point for smokers. Studies are limited[8,9] but suggest that acupuncture itself is ineffective for weight reduction and for cessation of smoking from a long-term point of view. Short-term benefits are not unusual, but there must be a higher-than-average placebo response in this sort of situation. The caring, the empathy, and the regular support of the therapist are probably the key 'medicines'. However, the rise of endorphins produced by ear acu-puncture, especially with point *shen-men*, may well, in part, explain a short-term benefit (Chapter 8).

SCALP ACUPUNCTURE

This form of acupuncture is even more modern, and indeed not based at all on traditional Chinese medicine. The principle is very simple: scalp areas and points overlying specific areas of the brain are described. These areas have their functions exactly as in conventional medicine. By treating the proper scalp points, the corresponding areas of the brain will be stimulated, and theoretically facilitate an improvement of function. It follows that scalp acupuncture will be used for neurological diseases, including cerebrovascular accidents and Parkinson's disease. I have no experience of this method but understand that it is widely used in China.

HAND AND FOOT ACUPUNCTURE

This is yet another specialist area of acupuncture distinct from the main channels. Various points are described on the hands and feet, corresponding to certain parts of the body, especially subject to acute pain. In fact, this technique is mainly used in China for acute pain – especially acute back and neck lesions. I have no knowledge or experience of this method but will mention four points on the dorsum of the hand which should cover acute low back and neck pain. These are in the spaces between the second and third, and the fourth and fifth, metacarpals, two distally and two proximally. Apparently, fairly strong stimulation is required, *deqi* is very painful and the patients often faint! If that does not put you off, by all means have a go!

OTHER FORMS OF POINT STIMULATION

Needling is the oldest form of acupuncture point treatment and still probably the most effective. Applying electrical impulses direct to the skin without needles has already been mentioned. Applying manual pressure (with hands and fingers) to points is becoming increasingly popular as little knowledge or experience is necessary and the method is non-invasive. A lot of massage techniques incorporate the use of acu-points, and, even in osteopathy, trigger areas are well recognized. No doubt all these techniques offer benefit; if one believes in the stimulatory treatment of trigger points, then this is not surprising, although the effect is probably not as powerful as needling.

One of the most exciting recent advances, is the use of a laser. This shows promise, as, theoretically, the proper 'depth' of treatment can be achieved without using needles, and yet can obtain the right quality of 'stimulation'. Much work needs to be done before being able to recommend its general use. In any case, the cost of the currently available laser machines is prohibitively expensive!

'ASHI ONLY' ACUPUNCTURE

Treating only the tender/trigger points in painful conditions is a method enjoying increasing popularity in the West. It is certainly simpler, and even more acceptable conventionally, but is *not* classical teaching. It remains to be seen whether this method is equally effective. Until this occurs, however attractive, it would be premature and unwise to advocate its practice to the exclusion of the principles of traditional acupuncture.

8
ACADEMIC CONSIDERATIONS

Having described the more practical aspects of acupuncture, due consideration must be given to the two questions: does acupuncture work? and how does it work? Many conventional doctors will prefer to read this chapter first in order to be satisfied, before even thinking about practising acupuncture. Not only do the concepts stretch conventional credibility, but also the treatment itself – how can the act of inserting a needle, without doing anything else, have any therapeutic effect apart from placebo?

The first point I would like to get across is that, although there is a clearly defined traditional basis to acupuncture, there is no conventional scientific explanation for its practice. We cannot, as yet, give any explanation for this system of traditional Chinese medicine, and this is one of the main stumbling blocks that stop a lot of conventional doctors even considering acupuncture. However, to a certain extent, we can show that it works, and this surely should make us strive towards understanding the traditional principles and attempt to find a scientific basis for acupuncture.

This chapter will attempt to answer the first two questions as far as is possible at the moment.

DOES ACUPUNCTURE WORK?

Most of the studies that have been done, and that can be conventionally accepted, are about the treatment of painful conditions. This is unfortunate, in a way, as we have few adequate tests of the efficacy of acupuncture in its pure traditional form: treating internal disease. In other words, the pure roots of acupuncture remain inadequately tested, and yet studies abound relating to a relatively small part of traditional Chinese medicine, i.e. the treatment of pain. This appears to be the wrong way round, but, on the other hand, one can understand how it has come about. Pain is much easier to measure and more acceptable to treat in the West. Some earlier studies have shown a beneficial effect of acupuncture on asthma[10–12] and migraine[13]. More recently, two small but very well constructed trials[14,15] compared acupuncture with 'sham' acupuncture in the treatment of chronic obstructive pulmonary disease and asthma respectively. They both showed a significantly greater benefit from 'real' acupuncture. There are also descriptive reports[16] on the treatment of systemic disease that at least start opening the door in this field.

In 1977, Mendelson[17] found a 60% success rate in the acupuncture treatment of chronic painful conditions. In 1978, Mann[18] reported a series of 1000 patients, 73% of whom showed significant improvement. A well constructed but small study[19] compared acupuncture and piroxicam in osteoarthritis, and found acupuncture to be superior and free from side effects. Another study compared acupuncture and steroid injection for tennis elbow[20]. This showed a 62% benefit with acupuncture and a surprisingly low 30% benefit with steroid injection (at three months).

It is interesting to review the studies that have compared random needling to needling acupuncture points. Many of these studies[21–23] showed no statistical difference between the two treatment groups, but this, in fact, is really not surprising. It is now well known that any noxious stimulus can attenuate pain elsewhere in the body through the mechanism of 'diffuse noxious inhibitory control'[24]. How, then, are we able to compare 'painful' stimuli? At the very least, large numbers of patients are required for a reasonable evaluation and this is not the case in the above studies. On a more positive side, two studies[25,26] did show a statistically significant increased analgesic effect with 'true' acupuncture. However, by far the largest and best study[27] showed a 70% response rate to true acupuncture, 50% response rate to random needling, and a 30% response rate to placebo. This latter placebo response is now a generally accepted rate applicable to pain relief in any therapy.

Less noxious stimuli were used as placebo representations in three studies[28–30] comparing acupuncture and placebo in musculoskeletal conditions and headache. These showed a 70–75% response rate to acupuncture and only 25% placebo response. Other earlier studies[31–33] also suggested that acupuncture has significantly greater effects on pain than placebo stimulation. Experimental work in animals[34,35] leads to the same conclusions.

Of those studies above which included long-term follow-up, the average duration of analgesia from acupuncture was six months. This is in keeping with one's impression in clinical practice with regard to chronic or recurring conditions. A well-constructed long-term evaluation of acupuncture (electro) showed a 74% significant response rate, maintained well beyond three months[4].

One of the greatest existing examples of the efficacy of acupuncture is its use in anaesthesia. It is used in up to 60% of both minor and major surgical operations in some Chinese hospitals with a 90+% success rate. The advantages are obvious but the major disadvantage is lack of muscle relaxation in major surgery. Both classical and ear acupuncture points are used but stimulation is more prolonged, using electrotherapy. Western visitors to China[36,37] have witnessed and attested to the efficacy of anaesthesia by acupuncture. This surely must be the most dramatic demonstration of the analgesic effect of acupuncture.

The field is wide open for large-scale studies on the acupuncture treatment of systemic disease. The limitations are obvious, however, not least ethical considerations. Patient acceptability is likely to become less of a problem, but there needs to be many more medical practitioners using this type of acupuncture who would themselves be able to compare acupuncture and conventional medical treatment. We have learnt and will continue to learn much from the Chinese, many of whose practitioners practice traditional Chinese acupuncture and conventional medicine side by side. In that respect they are ideally placed.

Another untapped opening is to foster a new co-operation between the medical profession and the lay acupuncturists (those who are properly qualified to practice acupuncture to a high and comprehensive standard). This would allow the undertaking of large-scale comparative evaluation studies.

Apart from clinical trials, the way forward will also depend on continued research into the scientific mechanisms of acupuncture. The next section will describe the present state of knowledge (or ignorance?).

HOW DOES ACUPUNCTURE WORK?

How acupuncture works is largely unknown! Theories abound, some backed by extensive scientific work, but I feel that these just touch the surface and are possibly just minor or secondary effects which do not explain the central core of the mechanism of acupuncture. Most of these theories relate to analgesia, and, therefore, in no way can they be applied to the concepts of traditional Chinese medicine.

Historically, besides acupuncture, methods of fighting pain with pain go back as early as the 4th century BC. 'Cupping' (which is still practiced in traditional Chinese medicine) was practiced in ancient Greece and Rome. This relied on creating a partial vacuum in an inverted cup held over the skin. Cupping is still used extensively in the folk medicine of southern Europe. Cauterization with a red-hot iron rod was a more vicious way of stimulation, as was rubbing caustic substances into the skin. Burning moxa directly onto the skin was, and still is, practiced. It is salutary to consider that compared with all these methods, acupuncture is positively civilized and luxurious!

This leads to the very crude theory of 'counter irritation'. Simply speaking, a sufficiently painful stimulus will lessen the perception of another pain. As mentioned before[24], this can occur by diffuse noxious inhibitory control, but this is only a very small part of the story.

A more sophisticated extension of this is the 'Gate theory' of pain relief as described and studied by Melzach[38,39]. This states that pain impulses travelling along the small nerve fibres are inhibited by impulses that pass along the large nerve fibres. He actually demonstrated[39] that acupuncture stimulates the large nerve fibres, and proposed that a physiological alteration of the substantia gelatinosa occurs when this takes place. More work was done by Lewith and Kenyon[40] to extend this theory, on both man and animals, to show that acupuncture exerts its analgesic effects partly through the selective excitation of efferent pain inhibitory pathways. Afferent neural transmission seems to be important in producing analgesia by acupuncture[41].

Another exciting advance was the discovery of 'endorphins': naturally occuring potent opiate agonists. Endorphin CSF levels were found to be raised after acupuncture treatment[42–44]. Subsequently it has been shown that the analgesic effects could be blocked by naloxone, a morphine antagonist[40].

Apart from the endorphins, many other substances have been found to be significantly raised after acupuncture. The 'enkephalins' are notable among these, and, interestingly, seem to be more in evidence using high-frequency electro-acupuncture[45]. Other released substances associated with acupuncture include serotonin[46] and ACTH[47]. The Chinese have experimented using two rats with a cross-circulation link[37], and found that acupuncture applied to one rat was effective in relieving painful stimuli on the other. The implication is that the humoral effects of acupuncture are likely to be more important than the neurological ones. In the acupuncture treatment of asthma, increased plasma levels of cuclic AMP have been found[48], and adrenergic facilitation has been suggested as one of the mechanisms[15].

It is likely that a combined neuro-humoral mechanism plays some part at least in executing the effects of acupuncture. Work in China[49] has suggested that there is a supra-spinal centre, stimulatable by acupuncture, that can inhibit viscero-somatic reflexes. Work by Soper and Melzach[50] proposes that the reticular formation in the mid-brain is likely to be a key area. Electrical stimulation of points within the reticular formation produces analgesia in discreet areas of the body and particular body areas may project especially strongly to some reticular areas.

The autonomic nervous system is almost definitely involved in the acupuncture treatment of non-painful and painful conditions[16,40]. As mentioned earlier, there is a paucity of backed information regarding the acupuncture treatment of internal disease but this situation is likely to change in the near future. Acupuncture is becoming increasingly used, and found to be efficacious, in veterinary medicine[51] and this will yield much useful information. Apart from anything else, the human placebo element is significantly reduced in animals! A close correlation has been found between 'trigger points' (as understood in the West) and acupuncture points[52], and this again should lead us to believe that there must be a scientific basis to acupuncture.

When we start to compare the more modern forms of acupuncture (ear, scalp, hand and foot) with other fringe disciplines that come under the banner of 'holography', we enter a completely new and untested field of theory. Holography is a Greek term that imagines the organism as a whole, graphically inscribed in a part of that organism. As applied to the so called 'microcirculations' of acupuncture, these parts are reflected topographically as points or zones within a circumscribed part of the body representing the various structures and functions of the organism. Nasal reflexology and iridology use the nasal mucosa and iris respectively, as their holographic zones. Studying the current theories behind these methods[53], it seems that biophysics is going to become increasingly important in the interpretation of the science of acupuncture. Ultra modern techniques of acupuncture ('Voll', 'Vega') encompass a concept called 'bioelectronic regulatory medicine'[54]. These rely on the notion that measurable electrical activity occurs on the acupuncture channels and points (and others), and is altered specifically in certain disease processes. Another more far reaching notion is that a specific electrical property can be measured in a homeopathic medicine, and even be transferred to an inert fluid such as spring water. All these concepts are just too new and untested (as yet) for us to consider in this book. They do, however, open a gateway to another theoretical approach which could prove rewarding.

I have a simple approach to the conceptual mechanism of acupuncture which I explain to incredulous patients when they ask, "How does it work?". A pathogenic stimulus (be it painful or otherwise) produces a natural defence mechanism that has two components: undesirable elements and desirable (healing) elements – the inflammatory response typifies these. When the undesirable elements are in excess, a pathological process continues. A minimal stimulus (e.g. acupuncture) that is similar to, but less intense than the pathogenic stimulus may produce a higher proportion of desirable elements, which will then be able to combat the pathological process. This is really a modified version of the principle of homeopathy – 'treat like with like', and, in many ways, resembles our conventional theory of immunization. It is interesting to note that homeopathy is practiced extensively in China (possibly more than acupuncture).

It is important to realise that acupuncture is not unique magic – it is just a certain sort of stimulus applied to a point. It has been shown that electrical stimulation, heat and a variety of other intense sensory inputs can produce similar effects to acupuncture[24]. Therefore, acupuncture should be seen as one of many ways of applying sensory input to the appropriate areas.

If nothing else, this chapter surely provides food for thought! The potential for further scientific research is enormous as we still do not know how acupuncture works. But after all – how does aspirin work? At least as far as pain relief, I hope I have demonstrated that it does work, and that the future for acupuncture is exciting. Above all, of all the studies mentioned in this chapter, none reported serious side-effects. They clearly demonstrated that acupuncture, in the right hands, is a *safe* form of therapy. How many conventional therapies can we say that of ? Even if one can show that acupuncture is at least as effective as conventional treatment in certain conditions, the safety aspect should provide a major impetus to the use of acupuncture.

9
FURTHER INFORMATION

This book is not intended to be a 'complete DIY guide to acupuncture'! I have only been able to give you the briefest glimpse into this immense subject, and, I hope, enough practical information to facilitate the practice of some simple acupuncture. At the end of this chapter I have suggested some further reading which looks at the wider aspects of acupuncture and should certainly serve you well as sources of further study. However, they are not 'beginners' books, and do not allow you, as a beginner, to take a simple line of approach as I have attempted to do.

Not only is there new (and confusing) knowledge to be learnt, but also much practical technique. In this situation, initial confidence is of paramount importance, aided by learning in a peer group setting. These aims can be met by attending a proper course. However, I hope that some of you, after reading this book, will feel able to go ahead and practice some acupuncture, even before attending any courses. However you do it, the quicker you get started the better!

COURSES

We immediately enter a world of controversy here. There are two sorts of courses on acupuncture which are poles apart. On the one hand, there are the purist, comprehensive and rather long courses that attempt to give a complete grounding in acupuncture. They are attended by not only medical practitioners but also lay personnel, more likely to end up practicing full-time acupuncture. At the end of such a two to three year course, a qualification is usually gained (British Acupuncture Association).

On the other hand, there are the considerably shorter courses (two or three *days*) run principally for medical practitioners. These concentrate on the bare essentials of acupuncture with more detailed teaching on the more GP orientated conditions, mostly painful. A lot of these offer practical 'hands-on' experience which is obviously useful in order to gain initial confidence.

The arguments between the two camps have been discussed elsewhere in this book. The purists claim that "a little knowledge is a dangerous thing". This would be true if there was evidence that 'mis-acupuncture' could do harm, but this just is not so. One of the essential messages of this book is that, with the provisos described in previous chapters, acupuncture is *safe*. Most, if not all, the readers of this book will not have the time to learn 'complete' acupuncture, and so would be denied the opportunity to practice a simple method of acupuncture if it were not for the 'weekend' courses (and this book for that matter!). It is probably evident that this book shares the same philosophy as that behind the short courses. An important point to realise is that these short courses are intended mainly for conventional doctors, whose knowledge and experience must count towards the ability to selectively learn and apply an unconventional discipline. After being initiated into acupuncture, some may wish to progress further in this field, and this is a different matter.

For those wishing to take a short course, I would recommend obtaining a list of approved courses from the British Medical Acupuncture Society (see below). These are held in various locations up and down the country and some are expensive.

For long courses, apply to the British Acupuncture Association (see below).

ORGANIZATIONS ETC.

Not surprisingly, the above controversies apply equally when we discuss the organizations representing acupuncture.

British Medical Acupuncture Society, 67–69 Chancery Lane, London WC2 1AF

The British Medical Acupuncture Society (BMAS) has medical practitioners only (mostly GPs) in its membership. Associateship is obtainable after proposal from two members and full membership offered after a minimum of one year's practice of acupuncture (at least four hours a week).

No qualifications are needed apart from the basic medical degree. An excellent journal is regularly published (*Acupuncture in Medicine*) and courses and meetings organized. Because this organization is for doctors of medicine only, it is the *only* one representing the rather special needs of conventional practicing clinicians, most of whom will practice acupuncture side by side with their conventional medicine. It is criticized for not having a qualification in acupuncture as part of its spectrum. One would question the validity of a qualification, based on the rather confused knowledge acquired, to practice what is probably a rather narrow part of the spectrum of acupuncture. Even those parts of the spectrum are not entirely standardized. It is early days yet. The society strives to find a scientific basis for acupuncture – as time progresses, the knowledge will increase and become clearer. The basic medical qualification ensures at least a minimum standard of clinical practice.

Council for Acupuncture, 10 Belgrave Square, London SW1X 8HP

The Council for Acupuncture is a national umbrella body with an agreed code of ethics which controls the undermentioned organizations. The BMAS is not a member of the Council. The Council recognize the various qualifications pertaining to its members bodies.

British Acupuncture Association, 34 Alderney Street, London SW1B 4EU

One of the main member bodies is the British Acupuncture Association which seeks status as an independent profession. Members must have medical training in a field other than acupuncture, and a minimum of one year full-time training in acupuncture. In ascending order of seniority, its qualifications are : Dip Ac., Lic Ac., B Ac. and Dr Ac.

Other bodies

Other bodies and their respective qualifications include:

> Traditional Acupuncture Society: M.T.Ac.S.
> International Register of Oriental Medicine: B.Ac.
> Register of Traditional Chinese Medicine: M.R.T.C.M.

SUPPLIERS OF ACUPUNCTURE EQUIPMENT

P.H. Medical,
16 Birch Close,
New Haw, Weybridge,
Surrey KT15 3JT

Acu Medic Centre,
101–103 Camden High Street,
London NW1 7JN

Harmony Acupuncture Supplies Centre,
19 Ashford Road,
London E18 1JZ

RECOMMENDED JOURNALS

Acupuncture in Medicine (British Medical Acupuncture Society
Journal)

Pain

American Journal of Acupuncture

FURTHER READING (BOOKS)

Lewith, G.T. and Lewith, N.R. (1980). *Modern Chinese Acupuncture.* (Well-ing-borough: Thorsons)
Mann, F. (1978). *Acupuncture – the Ancient Chinese Art of Healing.* 3rd Edn. (London: Heinemann)
MacDonald, A. (1982). *Acupuncture – from Ancient Art to Modern Medicine.* (London: Unwin)
Lewith, G.T. (1985). *The Acupuncture Treatment of Internal Disease.* (Well-ingborough: Thorsons)
Chaitow, L. (1983). *The Acupuncture Treatment of Pain.* (Wellingborough: Thorsons)
Mann, F. (1966). *Atlas of Acupuncture.* (London: Heinemann)
Paine, D.L. (1984). Acupuncture - *Traditional Diagnosis and Treatment.* (London: East Asia Co.)
Beijing College. (1980). *Essentials of Chinese Acupuncture.* (China: Foreign Languages Press)
Kenyon, J. (1985). *Modern Techniques of Acupuncture.* Vol.1,2,3. (Welling-borough: Thorsons)

Mann, F. (1974). *The Treatment of Disease by Acupuncture.* 3rd Edn. (London: Heinemann)

Mann, F. (1964). *Meridians of Acupuncture.* (London: Heinemann)

Jiason Yang (1982). *The Way to Locate Acu-points.* (China: Foreign Languages Press)

REFERENCES

1. Reilly, D.T. (1983). Young doctors' views on alternative medicine. *Br. Med. J.,* 287, 337– 9

2. Hayhoe, S. (1981). Why not consider acupuncture? *J. R. Coll. Gen. Pract.* 31, 624

3. Lewith, G.T. (1984). How effective is acupuncture in the management of pain? *J. R. Coll.Gen. Pract.,* 34, 275–8

4. Cheung, J.Y. (1985). Effect of electro-acupuncture on chronic painful conditions in general medical practice. *Am.J.Chin.Med.,* 13, 33–8

5. Stryker, W.S., Gunn, R.A. and Francis, D.P. (1986). Outbreak of hepatitis B associated with acupuncture. *J. Fam.Pract.,* 22, 155–8

6. Fox, E.J. and Melzack, R. (1976). T.N.S. and acupuncture – comparison of treatment for low back pain. *Pain,* 2, 141

7. Laitinen, J. (1976). Acupuncture and T.N.S. in the treatment of chronic sacrolumbagia. *Am.J.Chin.Med.,* 4, 169

8. Gillams, J., Lewith, G.T. and Machin, D. (1984). Acupuncture and group therapy in stopping smoking. *Practitioner,* 228, 341– 4

9. Sterner, R. P., Hay, D. L . and Davis, A.W. (1982). Acupuncture therapy for the treatment of tobacco smoking addiction. *Am.J.Chin.Med.,* 10, 107–21

10. Vlrsik, K. (1980). The effect of acupuncture on pulmonary function in bronchial asthma. *Prog.Resp.Res.,* 14, 271–75

11. Takishma, T. (1982). The bronchodilator effect of acupuncture in asthma. *Ann.Allergy,* 48, 44 – 49

12. Yu, D.Y.C. (1976). Effect of acupuncture on asthma. *Clin.Sci.Mol.Med.,* 51, 503–509

13. Loh, L. (1984). Acupuncture versus medical treatment for migraine. *J. Neurol.Neurosurg.Psychiatr.,* 47, 33–37

14. Jobst, K. (1986). Controlled trial of acupuncture for disabling breathlessness. *Lancet,* 22, 1416 –18

15. Fung, K . P. (1986). Attenuation of exercise-induced asthma by acupuncture. *Lancet,* 22, 1419–21

16. Lewith, G.T. (1985). *The Acupuncture Treatment of Internal Disease.* (Wellingborough: Thorsons)

17. Mendelson, G. (1977). Acupuncture analgesia - review of clinical studies. *Aust.N.Z. J.Med.,* 7, 642– 8

18. Mann, F. (1978). *Acupuncture: The Ancient Chinese Art of Healing.* 3rd Edn. (London: Heinemann)

19. Junnila, S.Y.T. (1982). Acupuncture superior to piroxicam in the treatment of osteoarthritis. *Am.J.Acupuncture,* **10**, 241–346

20. Brattenberg, G. (1983). Acupuncture therapy for tennis elbow. *Pain,* **16**, 285–88

21. Lee, P.K. (1975). Treatment of chronic pain with acupuncture. *J. Am.Med.Assoc.,* **232**, 1133–35

22. Mendelson, G. (1983). Acupuncture treatment for chronic back pain. *Am.J.Med.,* **74**, 49–55

23. Gaw, A.C., Lenning, W.C. and Shaw, L.C. (1975). Efficacy of acupuncture on osteoarthritic pain. *N.Engl.J.Med.,* **293**, 375–8

24. LeBars, D., Dickenson, A.H. and Besson, J.M. (1979). Diffuse noxious inhibitory controls. *Pain,* **6**, 283–327

25. Weintraub, M. (1975). Acupuncture in musculoskeletal pain – a double blind controlled trial. *Clin.Pharmacol.Ther.,* **17**, 248

26. Hansen, P.E. and Hansen, J.H. (1981). Treatment of facial pain by acupuncture. *Acta Neurochir. (Wien),* **59**, 279

27. Lewith, G.T. and Machin, D. (1983). On the evaluation of the clinical effects of acupuncture. *Pain,* **16**, 111–127

28. Junnila, S.Y.T. (1982). Acupuncture therapy for chronic pain – a randomised comparison between acupuncture and pseudo-acupuncture. *Am.J.Acupuncture,* **10**, 259–62

29. Jensen, L.B., Melson, B. and Jensen, S.B.(1979).The effect of acupuncture on headaches. *Scand.J.Dent.Res.,* **87**, 373–380

30. Macdonald, A.J.R. (1983). Superficial acupuncture in the relief of chronic low back pain. *Ann.R.Coll.Surg.Engl.,* **65**, 44 – 6

31. Chapman, C.R., Wilson, M.E. and Gehrig, J.D. (1976). Comparative effects of acupuncture and T.N.S. on the perception of painful dental stimuli. *Pain,* **2**, 265

32. Anderson, D.G., Jamieson, J.L. and Man, S.C. (1974). Analgesic effects of acupuncture on the pain of ice-water. *Can.J.Psychol.,* **28**, 239

33. Stewart, D., Thomson, J. and Oswald, D. (1977). Acupuncture analgesia - an experimental investigation. *Br.Med.J.,* **1**, 67

34. Pomeranz, B., Cheng, R. and Law, P. (1977). Electrophysiological and behavioural responses to noxious stimuli, after acupuncture. *Exp.Neurol.* **54**, 172

35. Sandrew, BB., Yang, R.C.C. and Wang, S.C. (1978). Electroacupuncture analgesia in monkeys. *Arch.Int.Pharmacodyn.Ther.,* **231**, 274

36. Lewith, G.T. and Lewith, N.R. (1980). *Modern Chinese Acupuncture* (Wellingborough: Thorsons)

37. Ko, E.K. (1973). Acupuncture. *J.R.Coll.Gen.Pract.,* **23**, 265 –72

38. Melzack, P. and Wall, P. (1965). Pain mechanisms, a new theory.*Science,* **150**, 971–979

39. Melzack, P. (1973). The neural effects of acupuncture. *Pain,* **1**, 357

40. Lewith, G.T. and Kenyon, J.N. (1984). The physiological and psychological explanations for the mechanism of acupuncture as a treatment for chronic pain. *Soc.Sci.Med.*, **19**, 1367–8
41. Looney, G.L. (1974). Acupuncture study. *J.Am.Med.Assoc.*, **228**, 1522
42. Akil, C. (1978). Increase of endorphin level after acupuncture. *Science*, **201**, 463
43. Clement-Jones, V., McLoughlin, L. and Tomlin, S. (1980). Increased endorphin levels in human C.S.F. after acupuncture. *Lancet*, **2**, 946–9
44. Han, J.S. (1982). Neurochemical basis of acupuncture analgesia. *Ann.Rev.Pharmacol.Toxicol.*, **22**, 193–220
45. Clement-Jones, V., McLoughlin, L. and Lowry, P.J. (1979). Acupuncture in heroin addicts - changes in enkephalin and endorphin in blood and C.S.F. *Lancet*, **2**, 380 –83
46. Cheng, R.S. and Pomeranz, B. (1979). Electroacupuncture analgesia mediation by endorphin and non-endorphin systems. *Life Sci.*, **25**, 1957–62
47. Malizia, E., Andreucci, G. and Paolucci, D. (1979). Electroacupuncture and peripheral endorphin and ACTH levels. *Lancet*, **2**, 535– 6
48. Feng, J.G. (1983). Change of plasma cyclonucleotide and corticosteroid content in asthmatics. *Shanghai J.Trad.Chin.Med.*, **7**, 26–27
49. Eh Shen. (1975). Supra-spinal mechanism of acupuncture. *Chin.Med.J.*, **1**, 431
50. Soper, W.Y. and Melzack, R. (1982). Stimulation produced analgesia – evidence for somatopic organization in the mid-brain. *Brain Res.*, **251**, 301
51. Janssens, L.A.A. (1986). Acupuncture therapy in chronic osteoarthritis in dogs. *J.Small Anim.Pract.*, **27**, 825–837
52. Melzack, R., Stillwell, D.M. and Fox, E.J. (1977). Trigger points and acupuncture points for pain – correlations and implications. *Pain*, **3**, 3
53. Schjelderup, V. (1986). Holography, biophysics and acupuncture. *Acupuncture in Med.*, **3**, 20-22.
54. Kenyon, J.N. (1985). *Modern Techniques of Acupuncture*. Vol. 3 . (Wellingborough: Thorsons)

INDEX